I Reversed My Diabetes

HAPPINESS Formula for Pre-Diabetics, Diabetics and Obese

Tabish Gill

01st edition 2023

Disclaimer

The information in this book is not medical advice and should not be treated as such. This book provides information based on the author's experience and research and should not replace advice from a qualified health-care professional. Always consult your doctor regarding your individual needs and before making changes to your diet, exercise routine, or any other aspect of your health regimen.

To My Cherished Wife

From the moment this journey began, you have stood beside me, your steadfast presence reminding me of our shared dreams and hopes. Your enduring patience, your unwavering faith when the path seemed strewn with challenges, and the love that has never dimmed or faltered—these have been my most potent remedies, more powerful than any formula or regimen.

Each step I took was anchored in your strength; each victory sweetened by the joy in your eyes. Your encouragement became the rhythm of my heart, and your belief in me was the wind beneath my wings. When the nights were long and doubts crept in, your reassuring whispers were the balm that soothed and fortified my spirit.

This journey, while embarked upon by me, was lit by your love, guided by your wisdom, and propelled by your unwavering support. This book, and every triumph it recounts, is a testament to our shared struggles, our combined efforts, and our undying love. Thank you for being my constant and my endless source of inspiration.

Charting a Course to 'GLUCOTOPIA'

Dear Reader,

Ever felt like you've tried every health trick in the book, yet nothing seems to bring those elusive results? Trust me, I've been there. I am Tabish, not just a nurse, but someone who's walked the challenging path of diabetes.

Amidst the storm of advice and countless medical opinions, I discovered a haven, a sanctuary I've come to call 'GLUCOTOPIA'.

What is 'GLUCOTOPIA', you ask? It's that golden state of health, where blood sugar levels are just right, where weight is managed, and where you feel in sync with your body. It's a place of equilibrium, of perfect harmony. And guess what? I didn't stumble upon it by accident. I designed a route to it, through what I proudly call the "HAPPINESS Formula".

This book, "*I Reversed My Diabetes — HAPPINESS Formula for Prediabetics, Diabetics, and Obese*", isn't just a collection of facts. It's my life's story, the challenges, the failures, and the eventual breakthroughs. Through its pages, you'll embark on a voyage, sailing through the complex seas of our relationship with food, the overlooked facets of insulin resistance, and the secrets the food industry might not want you to know.

But here's the thing: 'GLUCOTOPIA' isn't a destination, it's a journey. An ongoing voyage where you are the captain.

With the 'HAPPINESS Formula' as your compass, you can steer your ship towards health, balance, and yes, happiness. Or, you can let the currents take you elsewhere. The choice, dear reader, is entirely yours.

Life will throw its storms and calm days at you. But remember, even in the fiercest storm, with the right tools and mindset, you can find your way to 'GLUCOTOPIA'. So, are you ready to embark on this transformative journey? If so, let's set sail together, towards a brighter, healthier horizon.

Wishing you health, clarity, and endless joy on this voyage,

Tabish.

Contents

Chapter One

The Road to Glucotopia

A Personal Awakening

L ife is full of twists and turns, right? One moment everything seems bright and beautiful, but the next moment we find ourselves confronted with challenges we never saw coming. That's just how life works for all of us.

Let me share something called "Glucotopia." It's a place that resembles our world, where people are irresistibly drawn to the allure of sugar. They indulge in their treats without giving it a thought, blissfully unaware of the potential health storm brewing inside them. Sounds familiar, doesn't it?

You see, it's not just our craving for treats that poses a problem; it's also the way we eat in today's society. Fast food, processed meals, and excessive indulgence have become like an eating disorder that affects each and every one of us. Convenience and taste often triumph over nutrition, leading many down a path that leads to health issues—diabetes being one of the most prevalent.

Imagine feeling constantly tired throughout the day despite getting enough sleep at night. Your body feels sluggish. Your mind is foggy. No matter how much you drink, you can't seem to quench your thirst. This was how I felt—and this was a turning point that marked the beginning of my journey to comprehend and manage my body's glucose levels.

And you know what? I'm not the only one dealing with this. People around the globe are waking up to these health challenges. It's how we respond to our bodies' signals that really shapes our journey toward health. And that's where Glucotopia comes in—it's like a symbol for how we navigate the world of health and sugar.

I have a memory of a patient, whom I'll call Mr. Smith to maintain his confidentiality. He wasn't just any patient; his intricate medical condition significantly influenced my understanding of diabetes. Being a nurse, I see both the triumphs and the harsh realities of medicine. Despite Mr. Smith making progress, his complex condition weighed heavily on my mind. It wasn't just about diabetes being an issue; it seemed like this condition lay at the very core of many of his problems. So, I found myself diving into current research and discussing it with colleagues, desperate to grasp the extent of a disease that seemed to drive much of the suffering in the cardiac care unit.

It is unfortunate to say that Mr. Smith's health took a turn for the worse. Despite our efforts and the excellent care we provided, his body could not withstand the toll caused by the interconnected network of arterial disease, high blood pressure, and diabetes. This was devastating for both our team and me personally. Losing Mr. Smith was not just losing a patient; it was a loss that made me deeply reflect on my profession, my understanding of illness, and my role as a caregiver.

In that moment, I realized that I needed to be more than a nurse attending to symptoms and giving medications. I aspired to be an advocate for understanding the causes of diseases like diabetes and how they intertwine with other conditions such as heart disease.

Mr. Smith's story remained ingrained in my mind, inspiring me to delve into knowledge acquisition and share that knowledge with others. His kindhearted nature and the lessons I learned from caring for him have influenced my approach toward health care. Every patient has their story and behind every condition lies a human narrative. As health-care providers, we must endeavor to look beyond symptoms and comprehend the individual, and acknowledge that diseases like diabetes are not merely secondary ailments but intricate primary contributors to various health issues.

Diabetes can have serious effects on our body and can affect any organ. Some people with diabetes die, while some stay strong throughout the course of their illness. But one thing is for sure: uncontrolled type 2 diabetes has devastating effects on our body. According to a report by the Centers for Disease Control and Prevention (CDC, 2023), in 2021 cardiovascular disease was the leading cause of death in the US. It can be worsened by diabetes, which was ranked eighth among the causes of death. This highlights the importance of implementing strategies for preventing and managing these conditions.

According to the American Heart Association, 68% of individuals aged 65 or older who have diabetes pass away due to heart diseases, while 16% succumb to stroke. It is noteworthy that adults with diabetes are two to four times more susceptible to heart-disease-related mortality compared to those without the condition (Hajar, 2017).

These statistics emphasize the correlation between diabetes and heart disease, highlighting the importance of effectively managing diabetes in order to mitigate the risk of developing complications related to the heart.

As time passed by, I found myself constantly haunted by memories of my patient's demise. I couldn't help but ponder if there was anything I could have done to avert such a tragic outcome. It took a couple of years for me to truly grasp the gravity of my situation when I started experiencing symptoms myself.

The demanding nature and long hours of my work would often leave me exhausted. Although caring for patients and ensuring their comfort and safety brought me joy, recently something felt amiss. I noticed a fatigue that didn't seem consistent with my busy lifestyle and lengthy workday.

Initially, I attributed this fatigue merely to being occupied with nursing duties, which is undeniably demanding work. As time passed and my work hours kept increasing, I noticed that my symptoms were getting worse. I started experiencing dizziness and feeling lightheaded while also finding it increasingly challenging to concentrate.

It was at this point that I realized something was not right. I couldn't ignore my symptoms any longer. I knew it was time to take action. Although initially hesitant about seeking help, I eventually came to the conclusion that it would be beneficial for me. After undergoing a series of tests, the results were shocking: I was diagnosed with type 2 diabetes.

Similar to people in Glucotopia, my first encounter with diabetes wasn't a realization but rather an unexpected and unsettling confrontation. It happened on a day filled with activities and occasional indulgences in sweet treats or so-called healthy food. However, during a checkup, everything changed dramatically.

The diagnosis hit me like a bolt out of the blue. At first, disbelief and denial consumed me. Words like "blood sugar," "insulin," and "HbA1c" swirled around me like confusing jargon. I found myself lost amid a sea of terminology, nutritional information, and lifestyle recommendations as I desperately tried to comprehend it all.

As I struggled to come to terms with my reality, a flood of questions overwhelmed me: "How did I end up in this situation?" "What mistakes did I make?" and "Is this all my fault?" The questions seemed never-ending. The comforting illusion of Glucotopia shattered, exposing a reality that was hard to accept.

The moment I realized what had happened, fear and panic took hold of me. I envisioned all sorts of consequences that could arise from this illness. Blindness, amputations, heart disease, and even premature death were among the distressing possibilities that came to mind.

With my heart pounding and my thoughts racing through potential scenarios, I hurried toward the glucometer to confirm the diagnosis and test my blood sugar levels. I was surrounded by astonished colleagues, who witnessed my alarming test result of 20 mmol/L blood glucose! For comparison, the normal range is between 3.9 mmol/L and 5.6 mmol/L.

At that moment, the cold strip of the glucometer felt like a condemning verdict, while the digital numbers on the screen stared back at me, confirming the truth. My heart thumped against my chest like a drumbeat, each pulse echoing the reading of 20 mmol/L. How could this be?

The hustle and bustle of my surroundings slowly faded away, becoming a hum as my attention fixated on that damning number. I could hear whispers among my colleagues, their shock permeating the air around me, although I felt disconnected from it all, as if observing the scene from a vantage point.

Time seemed to both stretch and contract. I understood what this signified—I had unknowingly become a resident of Glucotopia, a city that had once seemed blooming. Now, more than ever, I needed to dissect this city's secrets and expose its insidious mechanisms. In a twist of fate, I had become living proof of Glucotopia's deception—a realization that further reinforced my resolve. The time had come to wage war against this paradise and reclaim our inheritance of true health.

The next few days were a whirlwind of tests, discussions, and consultations. There were countless pills, injections, meal plans, and words of consolation. The world of Glucotopia, once an abstract concept I had often talked about, had now become my tangible reality, and it was just as relentless as I had warned my patients. But amid this tornado of shock and change, I found solace in my mission, my resolve becoming my anchor.

I started to observe Glucotopia, the city I was in, taking note of its ways, its challenges, and its allure. I analyzed my interactions with the city, examining every blood sugar spike, each craving, and even the subtle shifts in my mood, energy levels, and overall well-being. It was like conducting a personal case study where I experienced firsthand the tolls that this deceptive city took on me.

In my pursuit of health, I initially focused on portion control as the foundation of my dietary transformation. With unwavering determination, I dramatically reduced my food intake by 50%, convinced that this simple adjustment would set me on a path to recovery. Fresh juices became an essential for me, along with a serving of salad topped with my so-called healthy dressings. Four days a week were dedicated to exercise routines. It marked a beginning filled with hope and potential.

Over time, I started noticing changes. My body responded positively to my newfound discipline. There were initial improvements in how I felt overall. The weight began to come off. My energy levels skyrocketed. It was incredibly encouraging, to say the least. However, I had no idea that, behind this facade of advances, I was caught up in a trap.

Without my knowledge, there were limitations to my approach. Although I made an effort to eat less, I didn't really focus on the quality of my diet. The foods I ate, even though I reduced the amount, weren't necessarily the best choices for my body. Despite following a healthy routine, there were still hidden toxins, additives, and processed ingredients in some of the foods that were impeding my progress.

As I reached a plateau in my journey, I started to sense that something wasn't quite right. Despite all my efforts, I noticed that my health progress had come to a standstill. It was frustrating. I found myself relying on medications just to maintain the progress I had made. If I slightly deviated from my diet by indulging in treats or having larger portions, I would have to double my medication dosage—a decision that, looking back now, turned out to be harmful.

Little did I realize that this repetitive cycle was actually doing more harm then good. By depending on medications to compensate for my choices, all I was doing was masking the underlying issues instead of addressing them directly. The temporary relief provided by increasing the medication dosage only acted as a Band-Aid solution that hid the problem that needed attention.

It became crystal clear to me that it was time to move past the limitations of portion control and adopt a different approach. It was crucial for me to reassess not the quantity but the quality of the foods I was eating and find those best suited to my body. It was essential for me to embrace nourishing foods that could genuinely support both my well-being and my healing journey.

As I explored the lives of those around me closely, I noticed a troubling pattern. People confidently claimed to follow a healthy diet and proudly spoke of their avoidance of food after the evening. However, upon examining their food choices, I came across an alarming realization: what seemed like a path to wellness was actually filled with pitfalls.

When I glanced at their plates, I saw an assortment of foods that appeared to be full of vitality. Beneath this facade of wellness there were hidden dangers lurking. Their "healthy" meals were actually packed with lectins, unhealthy oils, and sneaky preservatives that offered nothing more than a sense of nourishment. Lectins are proteins that have the ability to attach themselves to carbohydrates. However, while these properties help plants protect themselves in their natural habitats, they can sometimes lead to issues in humans. This is because lectins are resistant to breakdown in the gut and can remain stable in the acidic environment of the digestive system (Harvard T. H. Chan School of Public Health, n.d.).

Our society has unknowingly been led astray into believing that they are embracing wellness by limiting their evening meals. However, the truth is that these so-called healthy choices are far from what they seem. It's all an illusion—a mirage that perpetuates the myth of a nourishing lifestyle while quietly draining our energy and vitality.

Transitioning to my way of eating was challenging; I found myself longing for my indulgent snacks and sweets and feeling hungry all the time.

Despite giving it my effort, I struggled with managing my blood sugar levels. The fear of miserably succumbing to illness like Mr. Smith haunted me. I didn't want to rely on others or need assistance with tasks. My ultimate desire was to live a healthy life without any health complications.

That's when I made up my mind to dive deeper into the research, determined to find a way to overcome the challenges posed by diabetes.

In the field of medicine, a traditional treatment approach for managing type 2 diabetes focuses on regulating blood sugar levels through the activation of a key enzyme involved in decreasing glucose production in the liver. At first glance, this strategy seems practical and efficient, ostensibly circumventing the body's more complex processes. Yet, upon closer examination of this approach, questions arise concerning the long-term side effects and the broader implications associated with such a treatment strategy. It's a universal truth in medicine that every treatment comes with side effects, an inherent aspect of the delicate balance in health interventions.

Let's take melatonin as an example—a hormone that regulates sleep. It is released by our own body, but when we rely on supplements for an extended period, our body's natural production of melatonin can decrease. A continuous external supply disrupts the body's ability to produce this hormone independently, which can lead to dependence. This demonstrates how our bodies strive to maintain a balance called "homeostasis."

Homeostasis is crucial for survival and optimal functioning, as it represents a state of equilibrium among all body systems. Our bodies are intricately designed to sustain this balance by responding and adapting to stimuli.

However, using this kind of treatment for a prolonged period of time—despite their benefits—can potentially disrupt the delicate balance within our bodies. Long-term usage may lead to side effects that interfere with our body's ability to maintain its stability. It's important to acknowledge that the human body is resilient and constantly strives to restore equilibrium. However, the continuous external manipulation caused by medications might hinder our body's capability to regulate itself.

Safety concerns have arisen around some treatments for diabetes. In August 2022, one particular treatment drew scrutiny when investigations detected traces of a carcinogenic compound known as nitrosamine or NDMA. Despite these unsettling findings, regulatory authorities, citing potential shortages, have opted to maintain the availability of this drug, balancing current patient needs against the imperative for rigorous safety assessments (Center for Drug Evaluation and Research, 2022).

Shifting focus to the broader category of diabetes management treatments, it's notable that prolonged use of some therapies can lead to a decrease in the absorption of crucial nutrients. For instance, vitamin B12, an essential nutrient for neurological function and red blood cell production, may become deficient. The absence of adequate vitamin B12 can lead to a spectrum of health issues, including anemia, nerve damage, and cognitive concerns, thus potentially throwing the body's delicate balance into disarray (Medicines and Healthcare products Regulatory Agency, 2022).

Prolonged use of some diabetes treatments may lead to a rare but serious condition known as lactic acidosis. This condition is characterized by an accumulation of lactic acid in the bloodstream, which can upset the body's delicate acid-base equilibrium. Symptoms may include generalized weakness, increased respiratory rate, and abdominal discomfort. Individuals with renal impairments or other health issues that affect the drug's clearance from the body are particularly at risk (Blough et al., 2015).

Additionally, long-term therapy may be associated with gastrointestinal disturbances, such as diarrhea, nausea, and abdominal pain. These issues can adversely affect the body's fluid and electrolyte balance, leading to further systemic imbalance.

As I explored the treatment of type 2 diabetes, it became clear that current medical treatments are important for keeping blood sugar under control but they don't actually fix the underlying problem and these treatments comes with side-effects too. These treatments are essential for preventing the serious immediate effects of having too much sugar in the blood, but they don't get to the heart of what causes diabetes in the first place.

The real causes of type 2 diabetes involve a mix of things like our environment and/or our genes, especially our eating and exercise habits. These are the areas that need our attention. Right now, we mostly just use medicine to make the symptoms better. It's like putting a bandage on a cut but not healing the cut itself.

This realization sparked a desire within me—a desire to challenge the norms and explore alternative approaches that would restore harmony to my body without relying solely on external interventions. It was time to delve deeper and uncover the wisdom of our bodies, searching for methods that align with our design.

Chapter Two

Decoding Glucotopia

Kick-Starting Your Journey to Health and Freedom

Welcome to Chapter 2 of our exploration. Here we will delve deeper into Glucotopia, in a representation of your body when it's at its healthiest state and functioning in harmony. In Glucotopia, everything operates smoothly, with healthy blood sugar levels, abundant energy, and overall well-being.

Essentially, Glucotopia is like your body's "thriving place." It's where your cells are energized, your mind is sharp, your emotions are stable, and you feel in sync with life. This chapter serves as your guide to reaching Glucotopia. It's packed with strategies, insights, and actionable steps to kick-start your journey toward health and freedom. So, get ready for an adventure!

In our world, it's easy for our natural balance to be disrupted. Unhealthy eating habits, lack of activity, and chronic stress often contribute to conditions like diabetes. However, it doesn't have to be this way. Each one of us has the potential to create our version of Glucotopia—a paradise of health where our bodies efficiently utilize and regulate glucose.

This journey toward Glucotopia goes beyond preventing or managing diabetes. It's about achieving a state of well-being where we can truly thrive, embracing the energy, clarity, and vitality that come with balanced blood sugar levels. This journey is about empowering our health and making choices to support our bodies and overall wellness.

In the upcoming chapters, we will explore various strategies and habits that can guide you toward a state I've termed "Glucotopia". Central to this journey is the HAPPINESS formula I've devised:

H: Hydration
A: Activity
P: Pasture-raised meat and eggs
P: Plants
I: Inflammation-free and fasting
N: Nourish
E: Elimination
S: Sleep & Supplements
S: Stress-free & Sugar-free

While we will touch upon these elements throughout the book, a deep dive into the intricacies and nuances of the HAPPINESS formula is presented in Chapters 15 and 16. This approach ensures that as you progress through the initial chapters, you will gather the foundational knowledge that will prepare you for the comprehensive discussion in the later sections.

This isn't just a formula; it's a culmination of research, experience, and dedication to transforming lives. I encourage you to journey with an open mind, knowing that each chapter is a step closer to understanding and achieving Glucotopia.

Remember, embarking on the path to Glucotopia means committing to your well-being. It's a promise to take charge of your health and strive for balance and wellness. Whether you're managing diabetes or prediabetes, or simply aiming to improve your health, this book offers a whole range of tools and insights.

I'll be introducing some distinctive and creative terms that are purely fictional, so there's no need to search for them online.

In the animated city of Glucotopia, where every cell played its part, life was energized by a vital essence called Glucovita, known in the real world as glucose. This bustling metropolis, a microcosm within the human body, thrived under the meticulous care of the Insulinas. These guardians were the stewards of Glucovita, which in our world, we refer to as insulin, ensuring the city maintained its harmonious balance, akin to what we call homeostasis.

Outside the robust walls of Glucotopia, a dark force, named Resistulin, akin to what we know as insulin resistance, began to stir, casting a shadow of imbalance. The first sign of trouble emerged with the arrival of GutLeak, a counterpart to the real-life leaky gut syndrome. This cunning intruder breached the defenses of Gutguard, our body's gut barrier, planting seeds of chaos. This breach opened the gates to Sensi Foodius, analogous to food sensitivity in our bodies, transforming harmless elements into triggers for systemic Inflamorin, mirroring inflammation in our world.

As the city grappled with these challenges, the sneaky Lectonians, representing lectins, weaved their way through, binding with Glucovita and disrupting the delicate equilibrium maintained by the Insulinas. Glucotopia found itself on a precipice, its future oscillating between enduring harmony and potential disaster.

Within the cell-laden streets of Glucotopia, the alarm bells rang against the growing threat of Resistulin. Hidden adversaries, named Pestidia and Herbidia, symbolizing pesticides and herbicides, quietly contaminated Glucovita. Meanwhile, mysterious entities called GeMeOo, a nod to GMOs, sowed disarray in Glucotopia's orderly existence.

As the insidious Greasoil, representing unhealthy oils, surreptitiously replaced the balanced Omegatriad (echoing omega fatty acids), a wave of inflammation engulfed the city. The once vibrant heartbeat of Glucotopia now throbbed with a weakened pulse, as these unknown stressors, reflective of real-life challenges, drained the energy and spirit of its cellular citizens.Blue light, an agent of Resistulin, unraveled the city's sleep, severing their connection to the rejuvenating red and near-infrared light, compounding the decline. Ignorance, Resistulin's most insidious ally, crept through the population, making the once-clear enemy indiscernible.

Desperate for respite, the citizens of Glucotopia turned to common remedies, seeking solace in various widely-used Medicoles (Medicines). These provided a semblance of relief, offering fleeting respites that many clung to like lifelines. Yet, despite this dependence, the overall vitality of the city continued to decline, for these Medicoles provided only temporary alleviation without addressing the underlying malaise that afflicted the heart of Glucotopia.

The once ebullient energy that fueled Glucotopia faded, its cells now hostages to fatigue. The citizens, fraught with despair, found themselves only treating the symptoms, blind to the creeping decay that Resistulin propagated. Hope remained a flickering flame within the Glucotopian heart, a wish that Medicoles could turn the tide. But as Resistulin's grip tightened, the once magnificent city faced its darkest hour. The fight for Glucotopia's future was now a race against time.

Glucotopia's soul was not just against an external foe but an internal one; the true battle was for the citizens to recognize and rise against the unseen adversary that was slowly extinguishing the lifeforce of their beloved home.

In Glucotopia, the air once hummed with the vibrant pulse of well-being. But dark times had fallen. The treacherous shadow of Resistulin had begun to stretch its tendrils through the city's streets, turning the harmony of this once-thriving place into a delicate balance, teetering on the brink of chaos.

As the once-lush landscapes of Glucotopia withered, besieged by the malicious forces of Pestidia and Herbidia, and the ambiguous nature of GeMeOo products, the city's fate hung in suspense. Unhealthy Greasoils seeped into the very fabric of the city, and the silent, pervasive march of Inflamorin threatened to extinguish the city's spark.

The citizens, once a picture of vigor, now walked with a heaviness, as if the gravity of Glucotopia itself had intensified, burdened by fatigue and a weariness that dulled their senses. Blue light cascaded in torrents, disrupting their natural rhythms and casting a pall over their existence. It seemed that all would be lost to the encroaching darkness, a night unending, where the ignorance of the people was the most potent weapon in Resistulin's armory.

But in the depths of despair, a beacon emerged. His name was Tabius, an enigmatic figure whose aura emanated not from Glucotopia but from a realm of higher knowledge and profound truth. With a presence that cut through the disarray, Tabius spoke, his voice a thread of silver in the dark: *"You shall know the truth, and the truth shall set you free."*

Gathering the beleaguered citizens, Tabius illuminated the path once bright with health and prosperity, now shrouded in the shadow of neglect and decay. His words, steeped in the wisdom of the universe, sowed seeds of defiance within the hearts of Glucotopians. He spoke of cities lost to the same fate, consumed by the very ignorance that now clawed at their gates.

With tales of Fastinter, Organio, and Activito, Tabius painted a vision of a restored balance, a city reclaimed. The Omegatriad could be harmonized once more, the lights of red and near-infrared could be harnessed to rekindle the dwindling flame of Glucotopia's spirit.

As the message of Tabius spread like dawn's gentle warmth, the people began to shake off the yoke of complacency. They questioned, they learned, and slowly, they awakened. Armed with knowledge, they began the work of healing: detoxifying their lands from Pestidia, Herbidia, and the fallout of GeMeOo, banishing Greasoils, and embracing the regenerative power of light in its purest forms.

The heart of the resistance was the once-mighty Gutguard. Tabius rallied the citizens to its defense, for in its strength lay the health of Glucotopia. Together, they purged the city of toxins, Lectinos, and the alluring deceit of BeautiLux. Every step taken was a stride towards emancipation, every act of defiance a blow against the shadow.

Resistulin, however, was not blind to the stirring winds of change. The villain readied its counterstrike, determined to smother the burgeoning light of rebellion. Yet the will of Glucotopia was resolute, kindled by the spark that Tabius had ignited. The battle for their city, for their health, and for their very essence had begun. With truth as their shield and knowledge as their spear, they stood united, ready to reclaim the harmony that Resistulin had sought to destroy. The fight to free Glucotopia from the clutches of the dark had begun, and in the hearts of its people burned the undying hope that the truth would, indeed, set them free.

As the citizens tirelessly worked to restore the wall, Resisitulin took notice. Seeing the city he had taken for granted starting to fight back sparked a rage in him. He launched a full-scale attack on Gutguard in an attempt to weaken the Glucotopians' spirit.

However, the inhabitants of Glucotopia remained undaunted. Empowered by knowledge, they repelled Resistulin's assault with a defense that caught him off guard. Amid the battle, they continued their efforts to rebuild the wall, using Tabius's teachings as their guiding tools.

Against all odds, the Glucotopians successfully held off Resisitulin's onslaught. After what felt like an age, the city finally achieved a significant triumph against its oppressor. This marked a turning point in their struggle, reigniting their hope for the future.

With the taste of victory, Glucotopia experienced a rebirth. The people were revitalized, their spirits lifted by the belief that they could truly turn things around. Under Tabius's guidance, the inhabitants embarked on the mission of restoring equilibrium to their city.

A revolution was underway throughout Glucotopia. They phased out GeMeOos and Pestidia from agricultural products, opting for healthier alternatives. The citizens embraced a reset to mend Gutleak issues by consuming Biopros and maintaining a diet with an appropriate Omegatriad ratio.

To restore their rhythms, they replaced exposure to blue light with more natural sources of light. They understood the importance of keeping their internal body clocks in check for their well-being and used near-infrared lights to simulate sunlight. The immediate impact of these changes was evident. The people of Glucotopia experienced health and increased energy levels. Their food sensitivities started to decrease, Inflamorin started to wither away from their bodies, and their constant feeling of fatigue started to fade. The city started to regain its former vibrancy, filling the citizens with newfound hope.

Undoubtedly, the "great reset" was an achievement that showcased Glucotopia's resilience and the transformative power of knowledge and change. Although the city was still in recovery, undeniable progress had been made. Glucotopia was now better equipped than ever to face the challenges on its journey toward liberation.

Despite all the advances made, the enemy refused to accept defeat. They launched an attack on Glucotopia by using deceptive marketing strategies and promoting convenience via harmful products. Their intention was to make the Glucotopians forget their hard-earned knowledge and revert to their old habits.

The enemy flooded the market with alternative products, each one more enticing than the last. However, thanks to their awareness and informed mindset, the people of Glucotopia saw through these schemes. They stood strong against temptation and refused to be swayed.

Leading from the frontlines, Tabius played a key role in helping citizens navigate through this maze effectively.

In spite of the attacks, the people of Glucotopia remained unwavering. Their unity was their strength, their knowledge their weapon. They resisted the allure of quick fixes and superficial treatments, instead adhering to healthy routines that embraced balance and mindfulness. This approach included choosing foods closer to their natural form, engaging in activities that nurtured both body and mind, and fostering habits that supported overall well-being. By focusing on holistic health rather than temporary solutions, they fortified their defenses against the complex challenges they faced.

The final stand of the villain proved futile. The citizens of Glucotopia emerged victorious. They successfully defended their city against the onslaught, demonstrating that knowledge truly holds power. The city regained its vibrancy as its inhabitants restored their health and vitality. Glucotopia reclaimed its freedom.

As calm settled after the dust of the battle had subsided, a new day dawned upon Glucotopia. The citizens, once bound by ignorance, now moved freely in their revitalized city. The once decaying metropolis now pulsed with life as its cells brimmed with vigor.

However, Tabius knew that their journey was far from over. Knowledge and awareness were not stagnant; they were an ever-evolving voyage. He reminded the citizens of this fact, encouraging them to continue learning and growing.

The tale of Glucotopia is my narrative, an account of my quest to regain my well-being from the clutches of diabetes. This journey involved exploration, sifting through expert insights, drawing upon the work of esteemed health-care professionals such as Dr. Gundry and Dr. Jason Fung, and, most, importantly conducting numerous self-experiments.

This path I've embarked on has been far more than nights spent immersed in medical textbooks and scientific research. It has been an emotional journey, filled with moments of confusion and determination. It felt as though I was a detective unraveling a mystery to uncover the truths about my well-being and how to regain control over it.

During this exploration, I stumbled upon something that I now refer to as the "HAPPINESS" formula. It goes beyond being a regimen; it serves as my personal guide toward health and overall wellness. Now, with excitement, I want to share it with you—not as a clinical prescription, but rather as a trusted friend revealing a cherished secret.

As we continue along this journey together, envision this not as a lecture but as an intimate conversation between friends. Imagine us sitting in a room, savoring tea while I share not just factual information but also stories—lessons learned from experience, triumphs achieved, and obstacles successfully overcome. We will make the language of medicine tangible and relatable—something you can embrace, feel connected to, and apply in your life.

Throughout my journey, I have come to realize that my diabetes goes beyond being a medical term or a set of symptoms. It reflects my habits, choices, and relationship with food. It isn't simply a metabolic disorder; it serves as a wake-up call, indicating that my way of life is not aligned with what my body needs. However, the remarkable revelation is that I have the power to change it. I can take charge, make decisions, and essentially undergo a transformation.

Just as I found my path toward achieving harmony and well-being in my Glucotopia, you too can embark on this journey. The road to reaching such a state begins with understanding, compassion, and being open to embracing a new way of living. Shall we commence?

Chapter Three

Behind the Glossy Labels

Unmasking the Food Industry's Hidden Agendas

The Evolution of the Food Industry's Priorities

As we embark on this journey into the landscape of the food industry, one recurring theme will raise particular concerns: the prioritization of profit over health. This transformation did not occur suddenly; rather, it has been a determined process characterized by subtle shifts that eventually reshaped priorities.

Interestingly, despite our expanding knowledge about nutrition and well-being, the food industry seems to have taken a different path. Instead of incorporating this newfound understanding into their practices to create healthier and nutrient-rich foods, they often disregard these revelations in favor of maximizing profits.

This shift in focus is evident in several ways. The shelves are now filled with products that boast about being "low fat," "sugar free," or "high protein," without paying sufficient attention to overall nutritional value or ingredient quality. The addition of artificial flavors, colors, and preservatives has become commonplace, with these additives often overshadowing the real food components in the product.

The age-old saying "we are what we eat" has never been more relevant. Our bodies are nourished by the substances we consume. The nutrients present in our diet, such as proteins, fats, carbohydrates, vitamins, and minerals, play a role in building and maintaining our cells. When we consume quality raw materials, our bodies can function optimally. However, when these materials are substandard, the repercussions are severe and often irreversible.

The food industry of today has become skilled at disguising their products. Behind labels and persuasive marketing phrases lie hidden strategies aimed at enticing consumers to keep coming back for more—sometimes at the expense of their well-being. This is especially true for sugar and processed foods, which are frequently marketed as convenient, delicious, and even healthy options.

Unpacking the Three Culprits: Salt, Sugar, and Fat

In his book *Salt, Sugar, Fat: How the Food Giants Hooked Us*, Michael Moss (2014) reveals the calculated tactics employed by the food industry to create irresistibly satisfying foods. These tactics revolve around manipulating three ingredients—salt, sugar, and fat—to exploit our biological cravings and encourage consumption.

The outcome is a diet filled with huge amounts of added sugars, leading to a range of health complications such as obesity, heart disease, and, in particular, diabetes.

The World Health Organization (2015), along with other health organizations, has raised concerns about the negative impact of diets high in sugar on global health. One of the concerns is the contribution to the diabetes epidemic.

Surprisingly, despite these warnings the food industry continues to promote these sugar-laden products, especially targeting children and vulnerable populations. The result? A diet that is overloaded with added sugars, leading to a range of health issues such as obesity and heart disease, as well as a worrying increase in diabetes cases (Krans, 2019).

The "Health Halo" Illusion

One powerful tool employed by food marketers is the concept of a "health halo," which can significantly impact consumer behavior. This is particularly concerning for individuals managing diabetes and other diet-related diseases.

The term health halo refers to a bias where consumers perceive a food product as healthy, based on a health claim or attribute. For example, consumers might mistakenly assume that a snack is healthy simply because its labeled as "natural," "organic," or "low fat," without considering its actual content of sugar or other unhealthy ingredients.

A study by Fernan et al. (2018) provides evidence of this bias. The researchers discovered that consumers often associate claims or labels with health benefits, leading to misunderstandings about the overall nutritional value of a product.

From a marketing perspective, leveraging the health halo effect proves to be incredibly effective. Companies utilize this strategy to market their products as healthy alternatives, attracting health-conscious consumers and potentially fetching higher prices. However, from a health standpoint there is cause for concern.

The issue arises when the notion of a health halo causes consumers to overlook the composition of a food item. For example, a cookie labeled as "gluten-free" may still contain large amounts of sugar, saturated fats, and calories. Similarly, a yogurt advertised as "low-fat" might compensate for the reduced fat content by adding substantial amounts of sugars that impact the taste. In some instances, the emphasis on one health claim distracts consumers from considering vital nutritional details, leading them to make choices that do not align with their health objectives.

A Personal Insight Into Health Halo Deception

One day, as I strolled through the aisles of a store, my attention was captivated by a gleaming biscuit package that boasted being made from arrowroot flour, a well-regarded gluten-free ingredient. At first, I felt genuinely thrilled, as it appeared to be a healthy alternative gracing the shelves! However, my excitement didn't last long. Upon examination, it became apparent that this was merely a tactic for marketing purposes—a health halo.

Let's delve into the biscuits' ingredients:

Wheat flour: This first ingredient contradicts the product's claim of being lectin free. Wheat is widely known to be one of the sources of lectins, and it also contains gluten.

Sugar: This is a common culprit found in processed food items. Regular consumption of high-sugar products can lead to health issues such as obesity, diabetes and heart disease.

Shortening (vegetable, modified palm: Essentially, this is a trans fat, which are renowned for raising cholesterol levels and contributing to inflammation.

Arrowroot flour: On its own, this seems like a healthy addition; however, when combined with harmful ingredients, as is the case in this product, its benefits are overshadowed.

Glucose fructose: This is another term for high-fructose corn syrup (HFCS), which has been associated with obesity, diabetes, and heart disease.

Corn starch: This is often used as a filler ingredient, and can cause an increase in blood sugar levels.

Salt: Consuming high amounts of salt can contribute to high blood pressure and other cardiovascular problems.

Glycerol: While generally considered safe, consuming excessive amounts of glycerol may lead to health issues, including diarrhea, bloating, excessive thirst, nausea, vomiting, headaches, dizziness, hyperglycemia, mild laxative effects, irregular heartbeat, and confusion.

Baking soda: This is generally considered safe for consumption but doesn't provide any health benefits.

Soy lecithin: This is used as an emulsifier. Some individuals may be allergic or sensitive to soy-based products.

Diammonium phosphate: This one is frequently used as a leavening agent in food. Although generally safe in small quantities, it doesn't offer any health advantages.

Sodium metabisulphite: A preservative that can trigger reactions among those with asthma.

Natural flavor: This term lacks meaning and could signify various things. It does not necessarily indicate any health benefits.

Contains wheat and soy sulphites: This indicates the presence of potential allergens, specifically for individuals who are sensitive or allergic.

Basically, the product seemed to present itself as healthy by using terms, like "contains arrowroot flour." However, when you take a look at the ingredients, it tells a different tale. The biscuits contain sugars, potential allergens, and other additives. This serves as a reminder that we should always examine labels beyond their surface claims.

This scenario can pose challenges for individuals managing conditions like diabetes. If someone with diabetes spots a food product labeled as "sugar-free" but fails to consider its carbohydrate content, they may unintentionally consume more carbs than intended, resulting in an undesirable spike in blood glucose levels.

Therefore, recognizing and understanding the health halo effect plays a role in making decisions about food choices. It serves as a reminder to go beyond marketing claims and thoroughly examine the information provided for each product.

As people gain knowledge about these strategies, they can make choices and reduce the risks associated with diseases related to diet.

The Lure of Advertising

In today's world, we are bombarded with advertising messages every single day. Especially when it comes to the food industry, their marketing campaigns are designed to tempt and persuade us that their products are "healthy," "organic," "low fat," and "natural." These attractive labels can be quite convincing—but how much truth do they actually hold? Let's unveil the truth and examine the facts.

Furthermore, our relationship with food has significantly changed with the emergence of processed products. These items, packed with high amounts of sugar, unhealthy fats, and salt, are specifically designed for overconsumption. Unfortunately, while our health is suffering, the food industry's profits keep growing.

The Low-Fat Fallacy

"Low-fat" and "fat-free" foods stormed into the market with gusto. Initially, these products were hailed as the solution to combat obesity, heart disease, and other health issues associated with a high-fat diet. Consumers were thrilled by this prospect. It seemed like we could enjoy our indulgences without feeling guilty, as long as they were labeled as "low-fat" or "fat-free"—right? However, this illusion didn't last long.

To make up for the loss of flavor caused by removing fat, companies decided to add sugar, artificial sweeteners, and various unhealthy additives to these foods. Ironically, the products that were meant to protect us from obesity and diabetes ended up contributing to these issues. The "low-fat" era ironically heralded an unprecedented surge in obesity and diabetes rates worldwide. According to estimates by the World Health Organization (2020), global obesity rates have nearly tripled since 1975.

Organic: A Promise or a Gimmick?

Then came the wave of "organic" products, promising a healthier, pesticide-free alternative to regular foods. Unfortunately, the organic label has now become more of a marketing gimmick than an assurance of quality. With loopholes in regulatory systems, some foods labeled as organic may still contain synthetic ingredients. "Organically raised" livestock may have just barely scraped by the minimum welfare standards, far from the idyllic, free-roaming farm animals we picture.

This trend doesn't end there. Misuse of labels extends beyond sugar free to terms such as "all natural," "no artificial colors or flavors," "heart healthy," or even claims to being made with real fruit. These terms may seem promising, but in reality they often prioritize marketing strategies over actual health advantages.

Portion Size

The impact of the food industry on portion sizes is an aspect that has often been overlooked in discussions about eating habits and public health. However, this topic is worth exploring, especially when it comes to overeating and how it can lead to diseases like diabetes.

The way the food industry manipulates portion sizes greatly influences how consumers perceive what a "normal" serving should be. The food industry often presents larger portion sizes as the standard or even as a bargain (e.g., supersized meals at fast-food chains). This tactic encourages consumers to eat more than they might otherwise, leading to an increase in energy intake.

A study by Rolls et al. (2002) discovered that when participants were presented with larger portion sizes, they tended to eat more regardless of their weight status. The study's authors concluded that larger portion sizes contribute to increased energy intake potentially leading to weight gain and obesity. Excessive eating and obesity pose risks when it comes to developing type 2 diabetes. When we consume calories than our bodies can effectively utilize it often leads to weight gain.

Carrying excess weight, particularly around the midsection, can progressively impair the body's ability to use insulin effectively, which can lead to insulin resistance. This condition disrupts the normal regulation of glucose, causing it to accumulate in our bloodstream and giving rise to the elevated blood sugar levels that are the hallmark of diabetes.

Furthermore, continued overeating can place strain on the pancreas as the body requires insulin to regulate blood sugar levels. This increased demand for insulin contributes to the development of type 2 diabetes.

It is crucial to acknowledge that the food industry's practice of promoting large portion sizes as the norm has implications for public health. Consumers need to be aware of these tactics and fully grasp the significance of portion control in maintaining a balanced diet and preventing diet-related diseases such as diabetes. Promoting education regarding portion sizes and individual nutritional needs is vital to encourage a shift away from the belief that "more is better" propagated by certain sectors within the food industry.

Historical Health Blunders

Our history with regard to "healthy" eating has been a path filled with numerous mistakes and misunderstandings. It serves as a reminder of how nutritional science is constantly evolving and of the risks associated with unquestioningly embracing "healthy" trends.

Consider margarine, for instance. There was a time when margarine was seen as a more healthy substitute for butter. It was marketed as a smart choice for health-conscious consumers. Things have changed over the years. We now know that the trans fats present in margarine can actually increase the risk of heart disease, completely contradicting its claim of being "heart healthy."

Another example is artificial sweeteners. Initially praised as a calorie-free miracle that could satisfy sugar cravings without any health effects, they were later discovered to carry potential risks. Numerous studies have linked sweeteners to an increased likelihood of metabolic syndrome, type 2 diabetes, and even cardiovascular disease.

For example, in a study by Meng et al. (2021), the researchers conducted an examination and analysis of multiple prospective cohort studies. This comprehensive approach allowed for an investigation into the health implications of our beverage choices. The findings tell a story. Drinks loaded with sugar, which many people casually enjoy, were unequivocally linked to an increased risk of developing type 2 diabetes. Surprisingly, this connection remained strong even after considering factors such as obesity.

However, the repercussions extended beyond diabetes alone. The research also revealed a correlation between these sweetened beverages and an elevated incidence of diseases. Additionally, an undeniable pattern emerged: as consumption of these drinks rose, overall mortality rates also increased. Contrary to popular belief that artificial sweeteners might be a healthier alternative, this study suggests that they too are associated with similar health risks to their sugar-filled counterparts.)

It's time to reconsider that notion. These sweetened beverages, often marketed as healthier alternatives, pose similar health risks to their sugar-filled counterparts. The study clearly demonstrated a dose–response relationship, which means that the more we consume these drinks, the greater the danger they present.

This study serves as a reminder that should encourage individuals to go beyond the flavor and take into account the wider health impacts of their drink choices.

These instances from the past serve as lessons for our future. They remind us not to follow every trend or piece of nutritional advice that comes along. Instead, we should approach these choices with discernment, skepticism, and reliance on evidence-based information.

You may have heard the anecdote about a frog placed in a pot of boiling water. It goes like this: if a frog is suddenly put into boiling water, it will jump out, instantly aware of the danger. But if the frog is placed in cool water that is slowly heated, it will not perceive the danger until it's too late. The frog is cooked to death.

This parable eerily mirrors our situation with modern health, particularly with diseases like diabetes.

But here's something unsettling to consider: the food you eat today could potentially have lasting effects on your health in the future. It's like planting a ticking time bomb inside your body that's set to explode at some point down the line. The instant gratification of taste may come at the expense of your long-term well-being, with consequences that won't become apparent until later in life.

The same applies to HFCS, which is commonly found in sodas, sweets, and various processed foods. Although HFCS can enhance the taste of food, its long-term consumption has been linked to obesity, diabetes, heart disease, and even liver damage.

In their pivotal research, Malik & Hu (2015) delve deep into the intricate relationship between fructose intake, primarily from sugar-sweetened beverages, and its impact on cardiometabolic health. By meticulously examining the specific role of fructose, they underscore the potential dangers lurking within these popular drinks. Their findings shed light on how sugar, particularly fructose, might be influencing the rising tide of cardiovascular and metabolic diseases. The insights garnered from this study serve as a clarion call to re-evaluate our dietary choices and understand the broader health implications associated with the seemingly innocuous consumption of sweetened beverages.

So, how can we protect ourselves from this situation? How can we reverse this trend and reclaim our health? The first step is awareness. By staying informed about the harm caused by food products and the deceptive practices of the food industry, we empower ourselves to make better choices.

It's time to break free from the shackles of ignorance and set a new standard for our well-being. We will use the HAPPINESS formula in this regard: when shopping or eating, if a food meets the criteria of the HAPPINESS formula, we will buy it or eat it; otherwise, we will not.

Moreover, it is important for us to carefully read and understand the meaning behind labels. Just because something is labeled as "low fat" or "sugar free" does not necessarily mean it is good for our health.

In reality, such products often contain additives in order to compensate for the absence of fat or sugar.

It's about time we shift our focus from convenience and taste toward prioritizing health and nutrition. Although it may seem like a difficult task, the benefits are well worth the effort. Stay tuned as I reveal the secrets to leading a life supported by expert opinions, extensive research, and a proven formula for finding happiness!

All About Sugar

Ah, sugar—the sweetest poison! It seems to be hiding in every corner of our diets. It's not limited to desserts and sweets; it can be found in breads, sauces, dressings, and supposedly "healthy" fruit juices. This pervasive presence of sugar in our meals is one of the food industry's deceptive strategies with significant consequences for our well-being.

You might be surprised to learn that sugar is an addictive substance. Research has demonstrated that it can create a dependency, similar to drugs. So, whenever you reach for that cookie or fizzy drink, just remember that it might not be satisfying your hunger but rather fueling an addiction.

In this section, we'll explore how to identify hidden sugars in our food and uncover the tactics employed by the food industry to make their products more enticing. I'll also share my strategies for managing sugar cravings and integrating alternatives into your diet.

Embarking on this journey may not be a walk, in the park, but I assure you it will be well worth it. The key to regaining your health lies within your hands. Let's move forward together toward a future filled with improved well-being.

Let me take you back a few decades to when an infamous study called the Seven Countries Study came into the spotlight. It blamed fats as the culprit behind heart disease. This study was deeply flawed; however, it managed to capture the world's attention. Governments and health organizations then began promoting diets and food companies seized the opportunity by producing "low-fat" and "fat-free" products ("Seven Countries Study," 2020).

But here's the ironic part: these products weren't healthier. In fact, they were worse. Removing fat from these foods made them taste unpleasant. To compensate for this lack of flavor, guess what they added? You got it right—sugar!

In the upcoming years, scientists started questioning the fat crusade. Numerous high-quality studies emerged that debunked the notion that saturated fat directly causes heart disease. For example, a meta-analysis of 72 studies found no evidence that omega-6 and omega-3 polyunsaturated fatty acids affect coronary outcomes (Chowdhury et al., 2014). The authors also found no significant evidence that dietary saturated fat is associated with an increased risk of coronary disease. In another meta-analysis looking at the correlation between saturated fat intake and cardiovascular disease, the researchers concluded that there isn't sufficient evidence from prospective epidemiologic studies to support the conclusion that dietary saturated fat is associated with an increased risk of coronary heart disease or cardiovascular disease (Siri-Tarino et al., 2010).

Unfortunately, by then irreversible damage had been done. The "low-fat" dogma had deeply ingrained itself into our minds and our society.

What you need to understand, my friends, is that not all fats are made equal. Yes, there are bad fats: the trans fats, and the overly processed vegetable oils. But there are also good fats: the avocados, the olive oil, the nuts and seeds like sesame and flax. These good fats are essential for our body. They provide energy, support cell growth, protect our organs, and are necessary for nutrient absorption.

Now let's imagine a product labeled as "healthy," "organic," or "natural." You will probably come across these tags on items like granola bars, cereals, or fruit juices. It's easy to be lured into thinking that these products are beneficial for your well-being, but if you turn that package around and examine the label, you might be astonished by the amount of sugar it contains.

The food industry has mastered the art of concealing sugar in plain sight. They employ more than 50 names for sugar, ranging from dextrose and maltose, to evaporated cane juice and fruit juice concentrate. The result? Consumers often fail to realize how much sugar they're consuming.

Trans fats emerge as a consequence of hydrogenation process that transforms vegetable oil into fat. "Hydrogenated" or "partially hydrogenated" oils are terms commonly found on ingredient lists. However, what they fail to mention upfront is that these are actually trans fats.

The concern arises from the fact that trans fats can increase your "bad" (low-density lipoprotein, or LDL) cholesterol levels while decreasing your "good" (high-density lipoprotein, or HDL) cholesterol levels. This contributes to the development of heart disease, stroke, and type 2 diabetes. Unfortunately, it took decades for the harmful effects of these hidden enemies to come to light. Despite being banned in many countries, trans fats still manage to find their way into our food.

Our main adversary here is ignorance. By shedding light on these issues, we take steps toward reclaiming our health and well-being.

I distinctly remember first delving into this matter—it was like unraveling Pandora's box. Every label I examined and every ingredient I researched seemed to uncover a concealed threat. I must admit that at first it felt overwhelming. However, let me assure you that there is hope.

I can vividly recall standing in the supermarket aisle scrutinizing labels for what felt like ages, while my shopping basket remained almost empty. It seemed like every product I picked up contained some "danger" ingredient or another.

It was a moment of realization. I came to understand that I needed to make a transformation not for my sake but also for the well-being of those dear to me.

It was a step-by-step process. I started by making small changes, swapping out one product at a time. I stopped buying those fancy "low-fat" or "zero trans-fat" products, instead opting for natural, wholesome foods. I chose local produce over the imported, pesticide-laden fruits and vegetables. I started cooking at home more, and when I did eat out, I made healthier choices.

I also began educating myself. I read up on studies, talked to experts, and attended workshops and seminars. I learned how to read and understand food labels better. I realized the importance of knowing what goes into my body.

It's been quite a journey, and I'm still learning every day. But I can tell you this—it's been worth it. I feel better, healthier, and more energized—and, most importantly, I've managed to reverse my diabetes and reclaim my health.

Chapter Four

Insulin Resistance and Diabetes

The Unseen Battle

O nce upon a time in the land of Glucotopia, nestled within the kingdom of Cellville, a harmony prevailed among all the cells. They thrived on the sweetness of Glucovita, also known as glucose or sugar. The revered Insulinas, like gatekeepers, played their part by unlocking the doors of these cells and warmly welcoming glucose inside.

As time passed, an intriguing character named Junkius Foodius (junk food) made his way into Glucotopia. With his vibrant colors and enticing aromas, he wasn't an ordinary visitor. He carried with him a treasure trove of unhealthy substances—tempting treats tainted with pesticides, morsels containing lectin, and pots filled with unhealthy oils.

The innocent Glucotopians couldn't resist the charm of Junkius Foodius. They started indulging in his offerings without caution or realizing the chaos they were inviting into their realm. With each passing day, the influence of Junkius Foodius grew stronger, and it began to cause changes within the cells of Cellville.

The accumulation of substances from Junkius Foodius's treasure trove disrupted the cells. Intoxicated by his treats, these cells turned a blind eye to the gentle knocks from the Insulinas. As a result, they locked their doors tightly shut, denying entry to glucose. This marked the beginning of an era characterized by Resistulin—a condition known as insulin resistance—which cast a shadow over this thriving kingdom.

Reflecting Reality: Understanding Insulin Resistance

In our world, the tale of Cellville is not just a parable; it mirrors the reality within our bodies when we consume unhealthy foods and adopt sedentary lifestyles. Insulin resistance, similar to the Resistulin era in our story, occurs when our cells become less responsive to insulin. This hormone, like the Insulinas in Cellville, is essential for regulating blood sugar levels. When cells start ignoring insulin's signals, glucose accumulates in the bloodstream, leading to a host of health issues.

At this point, it's crucial to address a common challenge faced by many with diabetes: understanding what constitutes a healthy diet. The world of nutrition is rife with myths and conflicting advice, especially concerning diabetes management. In the upcoming chapters, we will demystify these concepts, breaking down the myths surrounding 'healthy' and 'unhealthy' diets. We'll explore what dietary choices are truly beneficial for those with diabetes, recognizing that individuals with diabetes have unique nutritional needs and lifestyles.

Each person's journey with diabetes is distinct, and there's no one-size-fits-all solution. We'll delve into how to tailor your diet to fit your specific health needs, lifestyle, and preferences. This approach moves away from generic advice, focusing instead on personalized strategies that work for you as an individual with diabetes. It's about transforming your diet in a way that supports your health and aligns with your new way of life as someone managing diabetes.

Understanding Insulin Resistance: The Real Challenge Beyond Sugar

Before we dive in, let's talk about insulin. Imagine insulin as a diligent traffic cop in the bustling city of our body, directing the flow of glucose to maintain harmony and balance. It is a key player in our body's metabolic orchestra, performs a trio of critical functions with precision and balance:

1. **Regulates Blood Sugar Levels**: Insulin helps cells absorb glucose, akin to directing traffic smoothly through busy

streets, ensuring blood sugar levels stay within a safe range..
When blood sugar rises, such as after eating, insulin is released to help cells absorb this glucose, reducing blood sugar
levels to a safe, stable state.

2. **Promotes Fat Storage**: Insulin also facilitates the storage
of fat. It's like a wise city planner, storing excess resources
(glucose) as fat in 'storage facilities' (fat cells) for future use.
This process is essential for energy management and reserves.

3. **Aids in Breaking Down Fats and Proteins**: In times of
'resource scarcity' (fasting or low blood sugar), insulin helps
break down stored fat and protein, providing alternative energy. This function is activated during periods of fasting or
when blood sugar levels are low, providing the body with an
alternative energy source.

Now, let's explore the core of our health journey: **INSULIN RE-
SISTANCE**. It's a complex condition, not just about sugar intake
but about how our body's cells respond to insulin. While sugar often
gets the blame in our diets, the real issue we need to address is insulin
resistance.

Understanding insulin resistance offers a revealing and often
eye-opening perspective on health. It's a shift from the usual narrative
that focuses narrowly on sugar as the main dietary villain. In reality,
insulin resistance touches upon a much broader canvas of metabolic
health. When insulin resistance occurs, it's like a key communications
channel in our body being jammed. This affects not just one, but
multiple essential functions:

1. **Blood Sugar Chaos**: With insulin resistance, this process
of sugar regulation function is disrupted. It's like having a
communication breakdown in our city traffic system, leading to traffic jams (high blood sugar) and potential accidents
(health complications). The cells become less responsive to
insulin, making it harder for glucose to enter. As a result,
blood sugar levels remain high in blood.

2. **Fat Storage Overdrive**: In insulin resistance, the body's
ability to properly utilize insulin for these processes is im-

paired. The body keeps storing fat even when it doesn't need to, akin to a city continuously building storage units without using them. This can contribute to obesity, especially abdominal obesity, and sets the stage for other metabolic disorders. It's an issue that transcends mere calorie counting, focusing instead on the hormonal regulation of fat storage.

3. **Impaired Fat and Protein Breakdown**: Insulin affects the metabolism of not just carbohydrates but also fats and proteins. This impairment means the body may struggle to break down and utilize fats and proteins effectively. This can lead to an imbalance in energy metabolism and nutrient utilization, further complicating the body's overall metabolic health.

4. **Hormonal Imbalances:** Insulin resistance disrupts hunger hormones, like a miscommunication causing the city's residents to believe there's a constant food shortage, leading to overeating. It is intricately linked to the balance of two key hormones: leptin and ghrelin.
Leptin, a hormone released by fat cells, signals to our brain that we have enough energy stored and it's time to stop eating. However, in the scenario of insulin resistance, this signal often gets muddled. Despite having ample energy reserves, our brain doesn't receive the correct message, leading to persistent feelings of hunger.
Ghrelin, known as the 'hunger hormone,' works in concert with leptin. Under normal circumstances, it prompts us to eat when our energy levels are low and decreases after we've eaten. Insulin resistance, however, can disrupt this delicate balance, failing to suppress ghrelin effectively even after food intake. The result is an ongoing sensation of hunger, regardless of how much we have already eaten.
This hormonal imbalance plays a crucial role in the challenges associated with insulin resistance. It perpetuates a cycle of overeating and weight gain, which in turn further exacerbates insulin resistance, creating a self-sustaining loop of metabolic disruption. This not only makes weight management increasingly difficult but also paves the way for more

complex health issues like metabolic syndrome, encompassing diabetes, obesity, and hypertension.

5. **Systemic Effects and Co-morbidities:** Insulin resistance has far-reaching systemic effects that extend well beyond glucose metabolism. This condition acts as a catalyst for a cascade of health issues, leading to various co-morbidities that compound its impact on the body.

   a. **Cardiovascular Health**: Insulin resistance is closely linked with a higher risk of cardiovascular diseases. It contributes to atherosclerosis, where arteries become clogged and hardened, increasing the risk of heart attacks and strokes. This is often compounded by associated conditions like hypertension and dyslipidemia (abnormal lipid levels in the blood).

   b. **Metabolic Syndrome**: This is a cluster of conditions including high blood pressure, high blood sugar, excess body fat around the waist, and abnormal cholesterol levels. Insulin resistance is a key component of metabolic syndrome, which significantly increases the risk of heart disease, stroke, and type 2 diabetes.

   c. **Liver Function**: Non-alcoholic fatty liver disease (NAFLD) is another common comorbidity. Insulin resistance leads to an increased accumulation of fat in the liver, which can progress to liver inflammation and potentially to cirrhosis.

   d. **Kidney Health**: The kidneys can also be affected. Insulin resistance can lead to changes in kidney function and structure, contributing to the development of chronic kidney disease, which further exacerbates insulin resistance.

   e. **Reproductive Health**: In women, insulin resistance is a major factor in polycystic ovary syndrome (PCOS), leading to irregular menstrual cycles, infertility, and other hormonal imbalances.

f. **Cognitive Function**: Emerging research suggests a link between insulin resistance and cognitive decline, including Alzheimer's disease. Insulin resistance may impair brain glucose metabolism and contribute to neurodegeneration.

g. **Mental Health**: There's an observed connection between insulin resistance and mental health issues like depression and anxiety. The exact mechanisms are still being explored, but this highlights the systemic nature of insulin resistance.

This broader understanding sheds light on why managing insulin resistance is crucial for overall health. It's not just about cutting back on sugar or carbs. It's about looking at the bigger picture of how our bodies process and utilize these nutrients. By addressing insulin resistance, we're targeting a root cause of many metabolic issues, not just treating symptoms. This deeper insight is key to a more effective and holistic approach to health and well-being.

Factors That Contribute to Insulin Resistance

There are various factors that contribute to insulin resistance. These include inflammation, stress, the accumulation of fat in the liver and muscles, as well as dysfunction in the mitochondria, which are responsible for producing energy within our cells.

Inflammation's Impact on Insulin Resistance

Have you ever noticed that there is heat, pain, redness, and swelling around a sprained ankle? These are all signs of inflammation. This is the defense mechanism of the body: The body is saying that a specific area requires attention, and the body is doing its best to repair it. But sometimes inflammation doesn't work in favor of the body, and the body responds incorrectly.

When we consume foods that aren't healthy, it is just like repeatedly twisting that ankle. Our cells become irritated and inflamed, which leads to a miscommunication between insulin and cells. This is where those complicated sounding substances like interleukin 6 (IL-6) and tumor necrosis factor alpha (TNF-α) come into play. They act as messengers that create confusion in the signaling process, making it more challenging for insulin to carry out its tasks.

The Connection Between Oxidative Stress and Insulin Resistance

Oxidative stress might sound complex, but it's something that happens in our bodies whenever there's an imbalance between harmful free radicals and protective antioxidants. Think of free radicals as little sparks that can cause a fire (damage) if not properly contained. Antioxidants are like the firefighters, putting out those sparks before they can cause harm.

When there's an imbalance— too many sparks and not enough firefighters—damage occurs. In the case of insulin resistance, this damage affects the proteins and lipids that help insulin signal the cells to take up glucose. It's like a broken telephone line, disrupting the connection.

So, what can you do about it? Well, there are ways to address these issues. By focusing on a balanced diet that includes foods packed with antioxidants—like fruits, vegetables, and whole grains—while avoiding any lectins, you can reduce inflammation and restore balance.

In essence, choosing the right foods is like giving your body the tools it needs to repair the sprained ankle and fix the broken telephone line. By understanding how these scientific concepts translate into your daily life, you can take active steps toward restoring balance and enhancing your overall well-being.

Mitochondrial Dysfunction

Impaired functioning of mitochondria in the muscles has a significant impact on the development of insulin resistance. According to a study conducted by Kelley et al. (2002), individuals with type 2 diabetes showed a reduced ability of their muscles' mitochondria to properly metabolize glucose and fatty acids. Additionally, they had lower levels of mitochondria in their muscles, resulting in decreased energy production. This inefficiency in utilizing glucose contributes to the worsening of insulin resistance. To improve both health and insulin responsiveness, it is recommended to incorporate regular exercise into your routine and maintain a diet that includes nutrients known to support mitochondrial function, such as B vitamins, coenzyme Q10 (CoQ10), and L-carnitine.

Other Factors

A research article by Savage et al. (2005) published in the journal *Hypertension* provides insights into the mechanisms underlying the development of insulin resistance. According to this paper, insulin resistance is a condition influenced by factors such as genetic predisposition, obesity, lack of physical activity, poor dietary choices, and the natural aging process.

A significant portion of the article focuses on exploring the relationship between inflammation and insulin resistance. Insulin resistance is closely linked to fat accumulation in the liver and the skeletal muscles. Because of fat accumulation, the insulin signaling pathway is disrupted by the actions of cytokines (inflammatory molecules). These cytokines, which are produced in higher amounts in obese individuals, interfere with glucose transport into the cells and promote glucose production in the liver. Such disruptions are central to the onset of insulin resistance, with inflammation playing a pivotal role.

Another study published in *Current Diabetes Reports* (Lovejoy, 2002) provides an overview of how different types of dietary fats influence insulin resistance. According to this study, not all fats have the same effect. While trans fats and saturated fats have been correlated with a risk for developing insulin resistance and type 2 diabetes, monounsaturated and polyunsaturated fats (found in foods like olive oil, avocados, and fatty fish) may actually help enhance insulin sensitivity.

The study goes into detail about how trans fats can cause inflammation and make the body less responsive to insulin. Eating saturated fats can also contribute to weight gain, which is another risk factor for insulin resistance. Conversely, diets that include plenty of monounsaturated and polyunsaturated fats as well as a balanced mix of carbohydrates and proteins can actually improve insulin resistance.

Understanding these nuances is vital when it comes to creating nutrition plans for people who have or are at risk for insulin resistance. By focusing on healthy fats and reducing trans and saturated fat intake, it's possible to manage—and even improve—insulin resistance.

This complex network of interconnected conditions emphasizes the importance of managing insulin resistance not just for preventing type 2 diabetes but also for maintaining overall health and well-being.

Implementing Dietary Changes for Managing Insulin Resistance

In our quest to navigate the complex world of nutrition and health, we often cling to the popular notion of what constitutes 'healthy' food. However, the reality is far more nuanced and sometimes counterintuitive. As we embark on this journey together in the pages to come, prepare for revelations that may challenge your long-held beliefs. The narrative of Glucotopia, our fictional yet insightful realm, serves as a metaphor for this exploration. Here, we'll dissect the intricate dance between glucose and insulin in our bodies, akin to the interactions of characters in our allegorical world.

Consider for a moment the foods that have been stamped with the 'healthy' label. Are they truly champions of our well-being, or could they be cloaked villains contributing to a deeper metabolic chaos? We often fall victim to marketing ploys and widespread myths, making choices that we believe are nurturing our bodies, while in reality, they could be subtly paving the path toward insulin resistance and its cascade of consequences.

In Glucotopia, just as the characters were deceived by the allure of Junkius Foodius, we too are often misled by food choices that masquerade as healthy options. These foods, potentially high in hidden sugars, unhealthy fats, or inflammatory agents, are akin to the trojan horses in our diet, undermining our metabolic health. The journey to understanding true nutritional value is fraught with misconceptions, but fear not, for this book aims to be your compass in the murky waters of dietary choices.

This transition from ingesting what we perceive as healthy, to the gradual build-up of insulin resistance, is both subtle and sinister. It's a journey marked by small, often unnoticed steps, each one taking us further away from optimal health. As we peel back the layers of dietary myths and misconceptions, we'll explore how everyday choices impact our body's insulin response. It's a story that unfolds in every bite, every snack, every meal. By understanding the hidden truths behind our food choices, we arm ourselves with the power to rewrite our health narrative, steering clear from the shadowy paths of insulin resistance and towards a life of vitality and wellness.

Diet plays a pivotal role in managing insulin resistance. The focus should be on reducing the intake of simple sugars and refined carbohydrates, which cause sharp spikes in blood sugar and insulin levels. A diet rich in fiber, lean proteins, and complex carbohydrates from whole grains can help stabilize blood glucose levels.

Emphasizing a balance of macronutrients—proteins, fats, and carbohydrates—can help in improving insulin sensitivity. Dietary adjustments should be personalized, taking into account individual health status, preferences, and cultural dietary norms.

Addressing Misconceptions: Medication Is Not a Free Pass

A common misconception in managing diabetes and insulin resistance is the notion that medication can offset poor dietary choices, allowing individuals to eat whatever they want without consequences. It is critical to dispel this myth and reinforce that while medications like insulin and oral hypoglycemics can help manage blood sugar levels, they are not remedies for unhealthy eating habits.

Medications are designed to work in conjunction with a healthy lifestyle, not in place of one. Relying solely on medication while continuing to consume excessive amounts of simple carbohydrates and unhealthy fats will likely lead to the accumulation of fat in inappropriate areas, such as around organs (visceral fat). This not only contributes to the worsening of insulin resistance but also increases the risk of other health complications, including cardiovascular diseases.

Understanding Insulin's Role and Its Misuse

As stated earlier, Insulin is a key hormone in regulating blood glucose levels, but it also plays a role in fat storage. When insulin is introduced into the body through medication, without the corresponding need due to excess dietary glucose, it promotes the storage of fat. Over time, this can lead to weight gain and a cascade of health issues that can "wreak havoc" in the future, as you aptly put it.

It's essential for individuals to understand that managing blood sugar is not just about the numbers on a glucometer or lab report; it's about the internal balance of energy and metabolism. The misuse of insulin or other diabetes medications to 'cover' for poor dietary choices is a dangerous practice with far-reaching health implications.

Incorporating Holistic Strategies for Health

In addition to the emphasis on healthy eating and the judicious use of medication, holistic strategies that encompass physical activity, stress reduction, and sleep management are equally important. These lifestyle pillars work synergistically to improve insulin sensitivity and reduce the need for medication, leading to a healthier future.

Targeting the Root – Overcoming Insulin Resistance

As we consider the challenge of maintaining healthy blood sugar levels, it's vital to shift our perspective from the immediate figures displayed on a glucometer to the intricate dance of hormones and energy within our bodies. Insulin resistance, the subtle yet profound defiance of cells to insulin's signal, stands as the true adversary in our quest for health. It is this resistance that we must diligently work to overcome, not merely the transient sugar spikes that are but a symptom of a deeper imbalance.

The strategies we will explore throughout the book aren't merely about lowering blood sugar levels; they are about reversing the conditions that give rise to insulin resistance. A holistic approach that includes dietary changes, increased physical activity, stress reduction, and appropriate use of medication is crucial in this endeavor.

As we close this chapter, I encourage you to harness this knowledge and convert it into daily practices. The path ahead is not merely about managing a condition—it is about reinvigorating your health and reclaiming the vibrancy of life. Let us march forward, armed with the power of informed choices and the resilience to adapt and thrive.

Together, let's look beyond glucose levels and focus on the ultimate goal: overcoming insulin resistance to lead fuller, healthier lives.

Chapter Five

Metabolic Disorder or Eating Disorder?

Unmasking the True Enemy

I n recent years there has been a focus on type 2 diabetes, which is widely known as a metabolic condition. Both the medical community and the general public now understand it as a disorder where the body struggles to use insulin, resulting in high blood sugar levels. While this disruption in our physiology is commonly attributed to genetics, sedentary lifestyles, and dietary choices, delving deeper into the disease reveals aspects that go beyond metabolism.

While the metabolic aspect of this condition is undoubtedly crucial, it's important to consider how our eating habits, our relationship with food, and even our emotional responses play a role. Could it be possible that what we primarily perceive as a metabolic disorder also exhibits characteristics of an eating disorder? The answer isn't straightforward; it's a conversation intertwined with psychological elements.

It's not uncommon to encounter diabetes patients who, in response to their diagnosis, vacillate between extremes of restrictive eating and bouts of indulgence, often secretively. The feeling of deprivation can lead to cycles of binge eating, only to be followed by intense guilt and further restriction. This cyclic pattern, reminiscent of certain eating disorders, raises an important question: is the physiological battle with blood sugar management inextricably linked with a psychological skirmish related to food and self-perception?

Moreover, the challenges presented by type 2 diabetes, such as glucose monitoring, dietary adjustments, and the constant worry about complications, often have emotional implications. These emotions in turn impact our eating habits. For some individuals, food becomes a source of comfort—a coping mechanism for turmoil—further blurring the distinction between metabolic disruption and disordered eating.

This chapter embarks on a journey to uncover these intersections and comprehend type 2 diabetes not merely as an anomaly, but as a condition deeply rooted in our mindset, behaviors, and emotions. As we navigate through this landscape, our aspiration is to achieve an empathetic understanding of type 2 diabetes by acknowledging its complexities and addressing it through a holistic approach.

Understanding the Basics

As we have touched upon earlier, insulin is a key player in our body's metabolism, crucial for guiding glucose into cells where it's converted into energy. If this process is compromised, it leads to a scenario where glucose remains in the bloodstream rather than being utilized effectively, which can be a stepping stone towards the development of type 2 diabetes.

While insulin resistance lies at the core of type 2 diabetes, several factors contribute to its progression from insulin resistance to full blown diabetes.

Lifestyle Choices

Sedentary lifestyles and diets high in processed foods, sugars, and unhealthy fats play a role. For example, consuming a high-sugar diet not only leads to high calorie intake but also causes blood sugar levels to rise rapidly. This puts strain on the pancreas, forcing it to produce insulin. Over time, this constant demand can make cells less responsive to the effects of insulin.

Genetics

Family history can play a role in determining one's risk for developing type 2 diabetes. If you have relatives with the disease, you risk is higher.

Certain genetic markers have been identified that make individuals more susceptible to insulin resistance. An article in *Current Diabetes Reports* (McCarthy & Zeggini, 2009) highlighted gene variants that could potentially increase susceptibility to type 2 diabetes.

Medical Conditions

Certain medical conditions, such as polycystic ovary syndrome (PCOS) or conditions requiring steroid medications, can further elevate the risk of developing type 2 diabetes. PCOS is a hormonal disorder affecting around one in ten women of reproductive age. It often leads to irregular menstrual cycles, high levels of male hormones, and cysts in the ovaries. This can impact a woman's fertility and is linked to increased risks of certain metabolic conditions. PCOS often includes insulin resistance as a symptom, which could act as a precursor to type 2 diabetes. A comprehensive review published in Endocrine Reviews (Diamanti-Kandarakis & Dunaif, 2012) presented evidence on how insulin resistance and PCOS are closely interconnected.

Let's take a look at the story of Rita, a 42-year woman who leads an inactive lifestyle and has a family history of diabetes. Without realizing it, she regularly consumed food and sugary drinks that contributed to her insulin resistance. When she was diagnosed with PCOS in her 30s, Rita's insulin resistance worsened due to the manifestation of the syndrome. If she had been aware of how her genetics, dietary choices, and medical condition interacted, maybe she could have slowed down or even prevented her progression toward type 2 diabetes.

When we dive into understanding type 2 diabetes on a metabolic level, we come to realize that it is not one single issue caused by insulin malfunction alone. It is actually the result of numerous factors that amplify each other and contribute to this metabolic disorder. It is crucial for everyone, especially those at risk, to comprehend this complexity if they aim for well-being.

The Connection Between Binge Eating and Diabetes

Binge eating is characterized by the consumption of a significant amount of food in a short duration, accompanied by a sense of loss of control. For those with type 2 diabetes, this behavior can have particularly detrimental effects. The never-ending craving for carbohydrate-rich foods leads to pronounced spikes in blood sugar levels, which can be challenging to manage.

What causes these cravings? Carbohydrates cause blood sugar levels to rise rapidly, providing an energy boost and often improving mood. In the short term this might provide relief, especially if someone's blood sugar is low. However, in the long run it disrupts the balance of blood sugar regulation.

There's an additional aspect at play here. People with diabetes often face restrictions and guidelines that can make them feel deprived. This sense of deprivation can eventually lead to episodes of binge eating as a way of "letting go." Afterward, guilt sets in. This often triggers binge-eating behaviors and sets the stage for another binge episode.

Type 2 diabetes isn't just about numbers on a glucometer; it's also intrinsically linked to our emotional state. Emotional eating, a behavior where food becomes a refuge from stress, sadness, or even boredom, can seriously impede glycemic control.

Another insightful study published in the *Diabetes Care Journal* delved into how the stress of managing diabetes, coupled with the effects of fluctuating blood sugar levels, could contribute to binge eating disorders among younger adults.

When considering the relationship between type 2 diabetes and eating disorders, it becomes clear that a comprehensive approach that addresses both metabolic dysregulation and emotional well-being is crucial. This serves as a message for health-care providers, caregivers, and those affected by diabetes to recognize and address the signs in order to embark on a journey toward genuine holistic health.

It's important to recognize that type 2 diabetes and eating disorders are not separate issues but interconnected conditions that can influence one another. This connection often begins with the metabolic dysfunction in diabetes.

When people engage in eating patterns like these, they unintentionally worsen their insulin resistance. It becomes a cycle: the metabolic dysfunction triggers disordered eating behaviors, which further worsen the underlying metabolic dysfunction.

Psychological Factors

While the metabolic aspects lay the foundation for this intertwined relationship, there are also other dimensions associated with a diabetes diagnosis that contribute additional layers to the complex issue of disordered eating.

At times, societal influences play a vital role. Our culture bombards us with messages about the "perfect body," "superfoods," and the "right way to eat." For individuals living with type 2 diabetes, these messages not only create pressure but also serve as a constant reminder of their perceived "failure" to conform. Over time, managing their condition becomes more challenging as they grapple with societal expectations surrounding appearance and diet. This can sometimes push them toward poor eating habits as a means of coping.

In our quest for truth, it's important not just to question the prevailing narrative but also to have the courage to look at things from a fresh perspective. This new viewpoint might be unsettling or even challenging. It's precisely this discomfort that can help us identify our adversary and reveal the underlying causes of the crisis.

So, let's engage in this exercise: what if we redefine diabetes not as a metabolic disorder but as an eating disorder? I understand that deviating from the established understanding may seem radical or even inappropriate. However, bear with me, because it's through thinking that we can make groundbreaking realizations and bring about transformative changes.

This change in perspective doesn't aim to oversimplify diabetes or diminish its metabolic aspects. Instead, it seeks to enhance our comprehension of the condition by looking at it through a lens that considers our lifestyle choices and behaviors, particularly regarding food consumption. It invites us to question not just the mechanisms behind diabetes but also the societal, cultural, and personal factors that influence its development and progression.

By reconceptualizing diabetes as an eating disorder, we are compelled to examine our relationship with food. This urges us to evaluate how our food choices, which are influenced by factors like convenience, emotional comfort, cultural traditions, and marketing tactics, contribute to the increasing prevalence of diabetes. It compels us to question the normalcy of our eating habits and acknowledge the possibility that these norms might be fueling a health crisis.

Essentially, this fresh outlook challenges the established norms and pushes us to think outside of the box. It highlights the connection between our eating behaviors and the growing occurrence of diabetes. Furthermore, it encourages us not only to delve into the physical and biological aspects of diabetes, but also to explore the behavioral, societal, and psychological dimensions of this daunting disease.

Remember that every significant shift in how we perceive the world starts with an idea—a perspective that disrupts prevailing beliefs. By considering diabetes as an eating disorder, we are doing just that: questioning standing paradigms, redefining the issue at hand, and paving the way for innovative solutions. It goes beyond renaming diabetes; it involves transforming our approach toward it.

This fresh perspective is not meant to be a destination but rather an essential milestone on our journey toward discovering truth. It serves as a foundation that can lead us toward gaining a better understanding of diabetes and equipping us with the knowledge to conquer this opponent. It may seem like an unconventional idea, but sometimes it's these unconventional ideas that hold the solution to common challenges—because when we dare to think, that's when we can truly bring about long-lasting change.

The Significance of Our Eating Habits

Our eating habits act as a reflection of the condition of our health and well-being. They form a line in our battle against various health issues, including diabetes. The choices we make at our dining tables, while grocery shopping, or when ordering food are often fraught decisions that require us to battle against marketing tactics, convenience, and ingrained routines. It is within these choices and routines that our silent opponent finds its weapons.

Take a look around you. Everywhere you turn, there are fast-food chains, sugary beverage companies, and factories churning out packaged and processed foods. This isn't a localized occurrence; it's a global trend. Driven by profit motives, these entities have profoundly reshaped our food landscape. This has played a significant role in fueling the widespread diabetes epidemic: they unknowingly aid our adversary, facilitating its advance by creating an environment that promotes unhealthy eating patterns and spreads diabetes.

It's not solely the environment that poses a challenge. Our personal eating habits, developed over years and even generations, also play a role. From consuming large portions and favoring processed foods over fresh produce, to indulging in late-night snacks or skipping breakfast—these routine behaviors contribute significantly to the issue at hand.

However, it would be oversimplifying matters to attribute all of the blame to our eating habits. It's crucial to recognize that these habits do not emerge in isolation but result from an interplay of various factors, such as societal norms, cultural traditions, economic limitations, and even emotional states.

Over time, these behaviors become deeply ingrained in our routines—so intertwined with our lives that we often overlook their impact. We become immune to the harm they cause, seeing them as just a part of life. This acceptance and normalization of unhealthy eating habits poses challenges in our battle against diabetes.

Essentially, our eating patterns, influenced by external factors and personal decisions, are at the heart of our fight against diabetes. This is where the enemy is most active, exploiting our weaknesses and perpetuating its dominance. However, recognizing this truth is the first step toward regaining control. For in our habits also lies our most potent weapon: the power to reverse the damage and defeat this enemy. But first, we must dare to challenge the norm, question our choices, and embrace the possibility of change.

When it comes to dealing with the pressing issue of diabetes, it's natural to feel overwhelmed, as if you're facing a challenging obstacle. However, I want to assure you that, despite the magnitude of the challenge, it is not insurmountable. In fact, we have the power in our hands to change the tide. By acquiring knowledge, implementing strategies, and demonstrating unwavering determination, we can not just improve our eating habits but also regain control over our health and overall well-being.

Transforming our eating habits doesn't necessarily mean going on restrictive diets or completely eradicating our favorite foods from our life. It is about developing an understanding of what our bodies require and providing them with nourishing and balanced meals. It entails creating an environment where healthy choices are readily available and appealing. It involves breaking free from unhealthy habits and embracing alternatives that promote better health.

The first step toward transformation is building awareness. This includes recognizing sugars in foods, understanding the consequences of excessive reliance on processed meals, and appreciating the significance of consuming balanced meals regularly. Developing this awareness empowers us by equipping us with information for making informed choices.

Following awareness comes the transition phase. This is where we apply the knowledge we've gained to our lives. It's when we start replacing unhealthy choices with healthy ones, gradually reducing our reliance on processed foods, sugars, and unhealthy fats. This phase may present challenges. It's important to remember that it's normal to stumble along the way. What matters most is staying committed and continuing to move.

The last phase is maintenance. Here we focus on ensuring that our new eating habits become a part of our lifestyle. It's about being consistent and avoiding falling back into old patterns. It's about building resilience against temptations and making a long-term commitment to our well-being.

Throughout this journey, it's crucial to be patient and compassionate with ourselves. Changing ingrained habits takes time. There will be obstacles along the way. However, with each change and healthier choice we make, we come closer to conquering our foe.

This battle isn't fought alone. There are professionals, community groups, and even apps and online platforms that can offer support, advice, and motivation. Utilize these resources, lean on them when the journey gets tough, and celebrate your victories with them.

My goal with this book is to be your companion on this journey. In the upcoming chapters we will dive into the specifics, understanding the "what," "why," and "how" of transforming our eating habits. We'll explore the significance of food groups, identify the culprits hidden in our diets, discover delicious and nutritious alternatives, and much more.

Always remember that every little step makes a difference. Each healthy choice you make accumulates over time, gradually breaking down the barriers of diabetes. By altering our eating habits, we're not just improving our health, but also revolutionizing our lives. Let's embark, on this journey together.

Chapter Six

The Hidden Role of Leaky Gut Syndrome

The Cracks in Gutville

Gutville: The Nutrient Metropolis Next to Glucotopia!

Picture a neighboring city of Glucotopia called Gutville, a center that handles food parcels known as GlucoBits and extracts the nutrients they contain. Similar to the customs department at an airport, Gutville plays a role in meticulously inspecting each GlucoBit and separating the beneficial nutrients from the harmful ones. This careful process ensures that only the highest-quality nutrients make their way into our bloodstream, which acts as the highway leading to Glucotopia. Like any border city, Gutville is surrounded by walls made up of epithelial cells fortified with tight junction proteins. These walls function as gatekeepers, preventing undesirable elements from entering while selectively allowing beneficial nutrients to pass through into Glucotopia. The seamless cooperation between Gutville and Glucotopia exemplifies the efficiency of our body's machinery. However, over time cracks started appearing in the walls of Gutville. The sealed junctions began to loosen, creating small fissures. Suddenly, unwelcome guests such as bacteria, toxins, and digested food particles managed to sneak in through these breaches in what was once a secure border. This influx of intruders caused confusion among Glucotopia's security forces, our immune system, leading it to react excessively. The outcome was a sequence of reactions resulting in health problems.

Understanding Leaky Gut Syndrome

This disruptive situation in Gutville reflects an often-underestimated health concern in humans" leaky gut syndrome, scientifically referred to as "increased intestinal permeability." While not classified as a disease itself, this condition can pave the way for a range of health issues. From autoimmune disorders and type 2 diabetes to food sensitivities and mental well-being problems, the implications of leaky gut syndrome are extensive. The turmoil unfolding in Gutville resembles the scenario of pouring engine oil into a car's fuel tank. Like our Glucotopia and Gutville, a car is an intricate system designed for precision and efficiency. It has compartments dedicated to the different types of fuel and lubricants necessary for smooth operation. There's a tank for petrol, a reservoir for engine oil, a separate area for coolant, and so on. Each substance serves its purpose and has its designated place within the car's system. However, if we inexplicably decide to pour engine oil into the petrol tank, we are inviting catastrophe. The car isn't designed to run on engine oil for power, and trying to make it do so would only result in a breakdownSimilarly, our body, a machine with an intricate design and sophisticated functions, has distinct compartments and specific mechanisms. The digestive system is specifically designed to process food, extract nutrients, and keep unwanted substances out. When these boundaries are breached due to leaky gut syndrome, it disrupts the functioning of our body's systems just like using the wrong fuel in a car.

Effects on Body Systems

The problems arising from leaky gut syndrome go beyond digestive issues. Just as using the wrong fuel affects a car's performance, leaky gut syndrome compromises our overall health. The consequences can impact the systems that operate within us. As we explore the implications of leaky gut syndrome further, we come to understand that restoring gut health is essential—just like using the right fuel for your car is an absolute requirement for smooth and efficient operation.

Similar to how we address any issues with our car to prevent breakdowns, it's crucial to take action in repairing a leaky gut. By making lifestyle adjustments, we can strengthen the walls of Gutville (our digestive system), ensuring that our body receives the proper fuel it needs for optimal functioning.

Leaky gut can be a culprit behind various chronic health problems such as inflammation, food sensitivities, autoimmune disorders, insulin resistance, and even type 2 diabetes. When unexpected invaders enter our bodies, our immune system responds by causing inflammation. Over time, this inflammation can lead to long-term illnesses.

In our bodies, the culprits causing the cracks in the walls can be a range of things: a diet high in processed foods, stress, lack of sleep, overuse of antibiotics, and certain harmful substances like lectins. The last one might cause you to raise your eyebrows, but recent studies have shown that lectins —proteins found in many foods, especially in grains and legumes—may disrupt the gut barrier function, leading to increased intestinal permeability. We will talk about nasty lectins in the next chapter.

It's not all doom and gloom, though. The great thing is that our gut lining has the ability to heal and regain its integrity. Following a balanced diet that's rich in nutrients and low in processed foods can help soothe the gut. Taking probiotics and consuming prebiotics are also important for maintaining gut health, as these products support the growth of bacteria in the gut and strengthen its barrier.

Lessons from Gutville: Glucotopians and Gut Health

In Gutville, the wise residents known as Glucotopians took steps to repair their gut walls. They became more selective about the types of foods they consumed, making sure to only allow in those that were healthy and beneficial. They even sought assistance from characters like Probioticus and Prebioticus, who played a role in maintaining the integrity of their gut walls.

Like the Glucotopians, we too need to pay attention to our gut health. Leaky gut is not an isolated issue but can have wide-ranging effects on our overall health. By addressing it, we can better manage and even prevent chronic health issues. Keep those gut walls sturdy and Gutville—and, indeed, your body—will thank you.

To understand how leaky gut contributes to diseases, we need to grasp how our immune system functions. Imagine this: you're one of the guards in Glucotopia, a member of the Immuno Squad. Your main duty is to safeguard the kingdom against threats.

One day, an unfamiliar object appears in your kingdom unexpectedly. Let's call it Invadicus for the sake of this story. Your squad, armed with sophisticated weaponry specially created for this object, launches a counterattack and captures the invader. This weapon serves as a blueprint, and is now stored in your arsenal, ready to be deployed if another invasion occurs.

This is exactly how our immune system works. The weapons created to counter Invadicus are known as antibodies. These antibodies act as "memory cells," which can identify substances and promptly initiate an immune response against them. This mechanism forms the foundation of how vaccines operate too. Vaccines introduce elements of viruses or bacteria (like Invadicus) into our bodies, enabling our immune system to recognize them as threats and generate antibodies accordingly. Therefore, if we ever come across the pathogens again later on, our immune system is prepared to swiftly fend them off.

Now, imagine if our Immuno Squad mistakenly treats friendly visitors to Glucotopia as enemies. This scenario mirrors what occurs when our gut lining becomes "leaky." Due to openings in the gut lining, large molecules that should not enter our bloodstream start finding their way in. This situation triggers our immune system to launch a defense, which leads to a harmful reaction from our system.

The modern diet we follow today is filled with processed foods and is lacking in diversity. This can make our gut more permeable, creating conditions for misidentifications and overreactions by our system. This "friendly fire" can cause harm to our health, highlighting how important it is to maintain a balanced diet to preserve the integrity of our gut lining and overall well-being in Glucotopia.

The Domino Effect: Broader Implications of Gut Health

Ongoing inflammation in the body can lead to many health problems. One significant condition associated with the gut is insulin resistance, which as discussed previously is a precursor to type 2 diabetes.

Think of it like playing Jenga, where each block represents a food. When the gut lining is healthy and strong, removing blocks poses no problem. However, if the gut lining becomes thin and permeable, removing one block can cause the entire tower to collapse. Suddenly, we find ourselves with a weakened digestive system, insulin resistance, and various other health problems.

The human gastrointestinal tract houses trillions of micro-organisms, collectively known as the "gut microbiome," which plays a role in maintaining health. An imbalance in this microbiome, referred to as "dysbiosis," has been linked to the emergence of leaky gut syndrome and various other chronic health issues.

Modern Developments in Insulin Resistance and Leaky Gut Syndrome Studies

Recent advances in gut health research have further underscored the critical role of probiotics in reinforcing intestinal barrier function. A comprehensive systematic review and meta-analysis conducted in 2023 delved into the impact of probiotics on this vital aspect of gut health. Analyzing data from 26 randomized controlled trials with 1,891 participants, the study revealed that probiotics significantly enhance gut barrier integrity. This improvement was evidenced by increased transepithelial resistance (TER), along with reduced serum zonulin and endotoxin levels, markers indicative of a stronger, more selective gut lining (Zheng et al., 2023).

Moreover, this analysis illuminated the anti-inflammatory benefits of probiotics. Participants receiving probiotic supplements showed a marked reduction in inflammatory markers like CRP, TNF-a, and IL-6, underscoring the role of these beneficial bacteria in mitigating inflammation within the gut. In addition to these effects, probiotics were found to positively modulate the gut microbiota. Specifically, the enrichment of health-promoting bacterial strains such as Bifidobacterium and Lactobacillus was noted, aligning with earlier findings on the importance of these bacteria in maintaining gut health (Zheng et al., 2023).

These findings reinforce the concept that a well-balanced gut microbiome, bolstered by probiotic supplementation, plays a pivotal role in not only maintaining the integrity of the gut barrier but also in reducing inflammation and fostering a favorable microbial environment. This serves as further evidence for the potential of probiotics in the prevention and management of various gut-related health issues.

A variety of factors can contribute to imbalances in the gut microbiome. including diet, stress, the use of antibiotics, and exposure to toxins. To support a healthy gut microbiome and reduce the risk of leaky gut syndrome and related health issues, it is crucial to incorporate high-fiber foods, prebiotics, and probiotics into your diet. Additionally, managing your stress levels effectively, minimizing exposure to toxins, and using antibiotics judiciously are useful measures you can take.

Insulin resistance has been associated with gut permeability without the direct influence of obesity in young adults. The lack of a relationship between obesity and insulin resistance was possibly mediated by the contribution of obesity to gut permeability. This finding suggests that gut permeability may be a potential independent risk factor for the development of insulin resistance in healthy obese young adults (Mkumbuzi, 2020).

A groundbreaking article published in *BMC Gastroenterology* marked a pivotal moment in our understanding of intestinal health and its far-reaching implications (Bischoff et al., 2014). The authors elaborate on the complex dynamics of intestinal permeability, also known as leaky gut, and the role it plays in the onset and progression of various diseases.

According to this research, the integrity of our intestinal barrier is more than just a mechanism to regulate nutrient absorption; it's a vital line of defense against harmful substances from the gut entering our bloodstream. In situations where this protective barrier is compromised, undesirable particles—including toxins, microbes, and undigested food particles—can leak into the body, triggering inflammation and an immune response.

This article also brings attention to the fact that increased intestinal permeability is not only a *symptom* of other diseases but actually plays a significant role in *causing* them. In simpler terms, having a leaky gut can be the root cause of various health problems, rather than just a secondary effect. The range of conditions associated with the gut is diverse, and includes disorders such as inflammatory bowel disease, celiac disease, mental health issues, and even obesity.

What is fascinating about the article is that it mentions the potential to target gut permeability for disease prevention and treatment. It suggests that by restoring the health and strength of our gut barrier, we could potentially prevent or improve these diseases. The proposition here is revolutionary, opening new doors for treatment strategies that focus on the health of our gut.

This perspective completely changes how we approach our well-being. It emphasizes the role that gut health plays in wellness and urges us to be mindful of what we eat and how our lifestyle choices impact our gut. Armed with this knowledge, we can be empowered to make decisions that bring us closer to achieving health and well-being—a concept akin to Glucotopia.

A further paper published in the prestigious journal *Gastroenterology* shines a light on the crucial role diet plays in causing and treating inflammatory conditions of the gut, including those related to increased intestinal permeability, commonly known as leaky gut (Lee et al., 2015).

This paper presents an argument for how our eating habits significantly impact the overall health of our digestive system. It suggests that our diet can be a double-edged sword; while unhealthy eating patterns can contribute to gut and inflammatory bowel diseases, adopting a healthy diet has the potential to prevent or even reverse these conditions.

This paper provides evidence linking specific types of food—particularly those high in sugar and unhealthy fats—to an elevated risk of gut inflammation and leaky gut. These foods are found to disrupt the integrity of the barrier, allowing harmful substances to enter the bloodstream. This can contribute to inflammation, which is a key factor in various health issues.

Conversely, the article also emphasizes how diet can be therapeutically beneficial in managing and treating gut-related health problems. Diets that are abundant in fiber, antioxidants, healthy fats, and other beneficial nutrients are proven to support health by strengthening the barrier and reducing inflammation.

The information shared in this paper emphasizes the significance of maintaining a healthy diet to take care of our gut health. It reinforces the idea that what we eat has an impact on our well-being. These findings make the concept of achieving health through Glucotopia more attainable, motivating us to adopt healthier eating habits as an integral part of our lifestyle.

Other research, like that carried out by Hou et al. (2022), shows that a disruption in the balance of the gt microbiota, known as dysbiosis, can lead to numerous health problems. This includes chronic diseases such as obesity, diabetes, autoimmune diseases, and even certain types of cancer.

For instance, harmful bacteria residing in the gut can generate toxins that cause inflammation and harm the lining of the intestine, leading to leaky gut. This condition results in increased permeability of the intestines, enabling substances like toxins and bacteria to escape into the bloodstream. This then triggers a response and systemic inflammation that may contribute to diseases.

Additionally, it is important to note that the gut microbiome plays a role in metabolic function. An imbalance in gut bacteria can influence how our body processes energy, potentially leading to conditions such as obesity and type 2 diabetes. The health of our system has also been associated with our overall well-being: the collection of micro-organisms in our gut can have an impact on our brain function and behavior. An imbalance in the gut microbiome has been connected to health conditions such as depression and anxiety.

Therefore, it is crucial to prioritize the well-being of your gut. A balanced diet that includes a variety of high-fiber foods, regular exercise, sufficient sleep, and effective stress management all play a vital role in maintaining a healthy gut microbiome. Additionally, incorporating probiotics and prebiotics into your routine can assist in preserving or restoring the balance of micro-organisms in your gut.

To summarize, focusing on gut health can be a strategy for both preventing and managing illnesses due to the significant impact of gut health on overall well-being. However, it's important to acknowledge that research in this field is still progressing and further investigation is necessary to comprehend the intricacies of the gut microbiome and its relationship with health and disease. Here's a list of foods you should consider adding to your diet for optimal gut well-being:

High-Fiber Foods

Including high amounts of fiber in your diet—from fruits, vegetables, and whole grains (preferably lectin free)—will support the growth of beneficial bacteria in your gut by providing them with essential nutrients. Fiber also aids in maintaining bowel movements and reducing inflammation within the system.

Prebiotics and Postbiotics

Prebiotics refer to types of fiber that act as nourishment for the friendly bacteria residing in your gut. These substances arrive in the digestive system largely intact, as they are resistant to digestion by human enzymes. Once they reach the colon, they undergo fermentation by the micro-organisms in the gut. This process promotes the growth and sustenance of beneficial bacteria.

Postbiotics are the substances produced by micro-organisms as they interact with their surroundings. These substances include enzymes, peptides, short-chain fatty acids (SCFAs) and other metabolic byproducts. They have various benefits for our health:

Inflammatory effects: Postbiotics can help regulate the immune system and reduce inflammation. For example, SCFAs produced by gut bacteria can have inflammatory effects in the intestines.

Maintenance of gut barrier integrity: Some postbiotics contribute to strengthening the gut barrier, preventing unwanted substances from entering the bloodstream.

Antimicrobial activity: Certain postbiotic compounds possess properties that can inhibit the growth of harmful bacteria.

Modulation of gut microbiota: Postbiotics help manage the bacteria in your gut by supporting the good bacteria and keeping the harmful ones in check.

Stimulation of the immune system: Some postbiotics enhance the body's immune responses, aiding in its ability to fight infections.

Anticarcinogenic properties: Specific postbiotic compounds have demonstrated their ability to inhibit tumor cell growth or induce programmed cell death (apoptosis) in cancer cells.

Metabolic regulation: Postbiotics such as SCFAs can have roles in regulating metabolism by influencing processes like maintaining blood sugar.

Nature's Prebiotic Pantry: Nourishing Your Gut with Fiber-Rich Foods

Chicory Root: People often enjoy chicory root for its coffee-like taste. It's also known to be a source of prebiotics. Around 47% of the fiber found in chicory root comes from a type of fiber called "inulin," a type of prebiotic that nourishes the healthy bacteria in your gut.

Dandelion Greens: If you're looking to add some crunch to your salads, dandelion greens are a great choice. They contain 4 grams of fiber per 100 grams.

Jerusalem Artichoke: You may have heard of Jerusalem artichoke by its names "sunroot" or "sunchoke." This unique vegetable contains 2 grams of fiber per 100 grams, and an impressive 76% of that fiber is inulin.

Garlic: Beyond adding flavor to dishes, garlic plays a role as a pre-biotic by supporting the growth of *Bifidobacteria* in our gut. Additionally, it helps prevent the growth of bacteria that can cause diseases.

Onions: Onions are not only delicious but also pack in a whole host of health benefits. They are rich in both inulin and fruc-to-oligosaccharides, which act as prebiotics, promoting gut health and strengthening our system.

Leeks: Leeks come from the same family as onions and garlic and share many of their advantages. These vegetables are high in fibers that contribute to maintaining gut health.

Asparagus: Another vegetable worth mentioning when it comes to prebiotics is asparagus. It not only offers prebiotic properties but also serves as an antioxidant-rich option for your meals.

Green Bananas: While all bananas contain high amounts of inulin, unripe (green) bananas stand out for their content of resistant starch—an element that acts as a prebiotic, with beneficial effects on gut health.

Apples: Apples contain a fiber called pectin, which nourishes the bacteria in your gut and helps reduce the growth of harmful bacteria.

Flaxseeds: These seeds are a source of fiber, including the type that promotes a healthy gut. They can be easily incorporated into various dishes and are simple to include in your diet.

Postbiotics

Postbiotics refer to substances released by probiotics, such as metabolic by-products or components of cell walls. These substances have shown benefits for health, particularly in relation to gut health. It's worth noting that research on postbiotics is still new and further studies are required to comprehend their effects and sources.

While many fermented foods contain postbiotics due to the fermentation process, the specific levels and types can vary depending on factors like the strains of bacteria used, the fermentation conditions, and the type of food itself.

Here are some foods believed to contain postbiotics:

Sauerkraut: This fermented cabbage dish has been found to be rich in postbiotics.

Kimchi: Similar to sauerkraut, this Korean dish made from fermented vegetables is considered a source of postbiotics.

Yogurt: Not only does yogurt contain probiotics, it also contains postbiotics as it undergoes fermentation.

Kefir: Kefir is a type of milk beverage that goes through fermentation and contains various types of beneficial bacteria and possibly other by-products of fermentation.

Kombucha: Kombucha is a tea drink that undergoes fermentation and is known for its postbiotic content, along with other potentially healthy compounds produced during fermentation.

Cheese: Some types of cheese—those that have been aged—are believed to contain postbiotics as a result of the fermentation process they go through.

It's important to consider that the amount of postbiotics in these foods can vary based on how they're processed, and heat treatment may potentially eliminate them. Therefore, it's consuming these foods in their unpasteurized state that may provide significant potential benefits.

Keep in mind that, while postbiotics may offer health advantages, it is crucial to maintain a balanced and nutrient-rich diet overall. Always seek advice from a health-care professional before making any changes to your diet, especially if you have any underlying health conditions.

Foods With Anti-Inflammatory Properties

Anti-inflammatory foods are those that can help reduce inflammation in the body. Chronic inflammation can contribute to health issues such as heart disease, diabetes, cancer, and arthritis. Here is a list of some foods known for their anti-inflammatory properties:

Berries: Varieties like strawberries, blueberries, raspberries, and blackberries contain substantial amounts of fiber, vitamins, and minerals. They also possess antioxidants called "anthocyanins," which exhibit anti-inflammatory effects.

Fatty fish: Rich sources of omega-3 fatty acids include fish like salmon, sardines, mackerel, and trout. These nutrients have potent anti-inflammatory properties.

Broccoli: Broccoli is abundant in antioxidants that aid in reducing inflammation.

Avocados: Avocados offer a source of heart-healthy monounsaturated fats, known for their anti-inflammatory properties.

Green tea: Green tea is abundant in antioxidants, which are beneficial in reducing inflammation and preventing DNA damage.

Mushrooms: Mushrooms like shiitake and portobello contain compounds that possess anti-inflammatory properties.

Turmeric: Turmeric contains curcumin, a compound known for its ability to combat inflammation.

Extra-virgin olive oil: Extra-virgin olive oil is packed with compounds that have anti-inflammatory effects.

Dark chocolate: Dark chocolate with a cocoa content of 70% or higher provides antioxidants that aid in reducing inflammation.

Tomatoes: Tomatoes are rich in vitamin C, potassium, and lycopene (an antioxidant with anti-inflammatory properties). Remember to remove the peel and seeds as they may contain lectins.

Cherries: Cherries are a source of anthocyanins and catechins, both of which actively fight against inflammation.

Vegetables: Leafy green vegetables such as spinach and kale are packed with vitamins and minerals that can help alleviate inflammation.

Citrus: Citrus fruits like oranges, lemons, and others are high in vitamin C—a nutrient known for its anti-inflammatory benefits.

My Routine

As someone actively focused on improving my gut health and reducing issues with my gut, I have developed a routine that incorporates various interventions and therapies. To align with my intermittent fasting schedule, I typically set my eating window from 11am to 6pm. Here's an example of what my routine looks like (remember, here I am just sharing how I incorporate gut-friendly products into my diet; we will go through my whole schedule in later chapters):

First Thing in the Morning

Upon waking up, I start my day by enjoying a glass of water mixed with squeezed lemon juice, inulin powder, basil seeds, and a pinch of salt. This ritual helps kick-start my digestion, invigorate my nerves, and create a nurturing environment for my gut.

Since regular energy sources like carbohydrates aren't part of my diet during this time, I choose to supplement with one tablespoon of medium-chain triglyceride (MCT) oil in the morning. This keeps me energized throughout the day. If you prefer, taking it three times a day can provide benefits by supplying energy for the entire day while also aiding in reducing insulin resistance. However, it's important to note that MCT oil can have a laxative effect if you take more than one tablespoon at once.

Breakfast

When it comes to breakfast, I opt for gut-friendly options, such as a smoothie made with plant-based protein, leafy greens, and a prebiotic fiber source like flaxseed or chia seeds.

I break my fast with two pasture-raised eggs, either boiled or made into an omelette. I also have some avocado chunks on the side. To accompany my breakfast, I enjoy a cup of black coffee. (Please note that if you have hypertension, it's important to limit your caffeine intake.)

Mid-Morning Snack

As a mid-morning snack, I like to have a serving of low-sugar, high-fiber fruits such as berries or an apple. This helps me maintain my energy levels while promoting gut health. Occasionally, I prepare a salad using romaine lettuce, onions, guacamole, and lemon dressing, which provides a crunch and tastes delicious.

Lunch

For lunch, I opt for a balanced meal that includes pasture-raised protein sources along with healthy fats and plenty of colorful vegetables. To support my gut health further, I incorporate fermented vegetables like sauerkraut or kimchi into my meals, as they are rich in probiotics.

Afternoon

After lunch, I take my supplements—which include zinc, and curcumin—to promote my gut barrier function and reduce inflammation in my body.

Dinner

For dinner, I focus on creating meals that are beneficial for my gut health. My dinner plate usually consists of wild-caught salmon as the protein source, alongside steamed or roasted vegetables prepared in various flavors. As a side dish option, I often include yesterday's basmati rice to complement the meal. Reheating cold basmati rice transforms its carbohydrates into resistant starch, a dietary component favored by the beneficial bacteria in our gut. This process not only enhances the nutritional value of the rice but also contributes positively to gut health by feeding the 'good' microbes residing in our digestive system.

Before Bed

Before I go to bed, I like to have a mug of herbal tea, such as peppermint or chamomile. This helps with digestion and soothes my stomach.

By sticking to this routine, I've managed to improve my issues with my gut and promote a healthy gut microbiome. However, it's important to remember that everyone's needs are different. Before making any changes to your diet or supplements, it's always wise to consult with a health-care professional.

The field of medicine now offers strategies and tools that can help us achieve better gut health when combined with lifestyle adjustments. Recent advances in technology and medical research have given us insights into our gut health. For instance, there are home testing kits that analyze our gut microbiota and offer personalized recommendations. Similarly, blood tests that can measure levels of zonulin—a protein indicating leaky gut when found in high concentrations—have become accessible.

Furthermore, treatments like fecal microbiota transplantation, an initially invasive procedure, have now been developed into oral capsules. Even more innovative are therapeutics directly addressing leaky gut syndrome, including drugs targeting molecules involved in gut barrier function and specially engineered probiotics.

Complementing these are mobile apps, which offer features for tracking diet, symptoms, and bowel movements, and innovative probiotics tailored to specific health needs. All of these, although still under study, represent a growing interest and optimism in the field of gut health.

Ultimately, while these advances offer exciting possibilities, they should serve to enhance, not replace, the core principles of maintaining a healthy diet, exercising regularly, ensuring adequate sleep, and managing stress. In Glucotopia, technology and therapeutics are valuable tools, but it is the choices we make every day that truly lay the foundation for health and well-being.

Chapter Seven

Lectins' Invasion

The Dangers Lurking in Your Food

T he storm that swept through Glucotopia and Gutville was a moment that provided valuable insights, which still resonate in these cities. One of the notable discoveries from that event was the existence of deceptive entities called Lectonians, known as "lectins" in our world. These sneaky substances can be found in various foods and, despite appearing harmless, they have the potential to cause havoc within our bodies and disrupt the harmony and well-being we strive for.

Initially disguised as nutrients, Lectonians managed to bypass the vigilant guards at Gutville's borders and infiltrated deep into the heart of Glucotopia. At first, their presence went unnoticed as they caused only minor disruptions that were easily overlooked. However, over time these insignificant disturbances escalated into widespread breakdowns throughout Glucotopia, resulting in internal chaos and unrest.

Lectins: Plants' Personal Security Team

Lectins are proteins that exist in plants and certain animal-based foods. They serve a role in safeguarding plants against pests and insects. To illustrate this, picture a caterpillar attempting to feast on a leaf; however, the leaf contains lectins that give the caterpillar a stomachache. As a result, the caterpillar is discouraged from returning for food, thus protecting the plant. In essence, for plants lectins act as their personal security team, keeping intruders at bay.

But here's the catch; While these proteins are great for plants, they can cause issues for us humans. Imagine them as a guest who wasn't invited but still showed up and caused a commotion. Our bodies struggle to digest them. When we consume large amounts of lectins, they can trigger inflammation.

The true danger of lectins lies in their ability to interfere with our body's communication systems by distorting vital signals that regulate our health. For example, lectins can mimic insulin, a player responsible for allowing glucose to enter our cells, which leads to confusion and contributes to insulin resistance—a major concern for Glucotopia. Insulin plays a role by ensuring a smooth flow of glucose to where it is most needed. Unfortunately, when lectins engage in their behavior, this delicate balance is disrupted. Impersonating insulin, lectins create confusion, making our body's cells resist genuine insulin. This leaves the gateways to the cells puzzled, uncertain whether to open or close. Consequently, Glucotopia faces a crisis: insulin resistance.

Understanding lectins and their cunning strategies is essential for preserving the health and integrity of our cities. It plays a role in our journey toward creating a flourishing Glucotopia, where problems like insulin resistance and high blood sugar are things of the past. By being mindful of lectins in our diet and managing our intake wisely, we can ensure operations within our bodily cities while supporting our quest for optimal health.

Practical Steps to Limit Lectin Intake

Similar to the enlightened residents of Glucotopia, we too can make informed choices to limit our intake of lectins. Although completely eliminating them from our diet may be challenging, we can certainly minimize their impact. Cooking, fermenting, and pressure-cooking are methods that reduce the levels of these disruptive agents in our food, restoring peace and balance within our bodies.

Just as Glucotopia and Gutville adapted and protected themselves from the lectin threat, we too have the opportunity to make choices that support our well being. The choices we make regarding our diet and food preparation can have an impact on maintaining a healthy gut. This in turn strengthens our body's defense against the risks associated with lectins.

Personal Reflections on Diet and Lectins

I can't help but look back at my own life and the eating habits I was accustomed to. Who would have guessed that my beloved childhood snack—a peanut butter sandwich, which seemed harmless—contained these tricky lectins? It wasn't just the sandwich: legumes like lentils and chickpeas, which are common ingredients in many traditional dishes, are also high in these compounds. I remember enjoying a bowl of lentil soup during the winter, savoring each spoonful without realizing the presence of hidden lectins.

I therefore began turning to the popular "superfood" quinoa. Mixed with vegetables, this became my go-to salad for a quick lunch. Little did I know then that even quinoa, as healthy as it sounds, is actually a significant source of lectins.

And it's not just me; we should consider our collective eating habits too. Wheat, an ingredient found in many staple foods across the globe, is known to contain lectins. Soy, which is frequently used in processed foods and vegan diets, is also a source of lectins.

It's important to note that my intention here is not to create fear or discourage the consumption of these foods. I still enjoy including legumes in my diet, and occasionally have quinoa salads. The main idea is to be mindful of what we eat, understand its impact on our bodies, and make informed choices about our diet.

Our bodies are truly incredible when it comes to adapting and recovering. However, they also rely on us to make decisions that support our well-being. This realization led me on a journey toward making conscious changes in my eating habits.

This transformation didn't happen overnight; instead, I started by making adjustments and gradually reducing my intake of high-lectin foods—those sneaky lectins that had been causing trouble in my Glucotopia. It wasn't always easy, since many of these foods were ones I used to enjoy and considered beneficial. Nevertheless, I was determined to help restore my body's balance and improve its health.

As I replaced high-lectin foods with alternatives each day, I began noticing tangible differences within myself. It felt like a haze was lifting and Glucotopia was getting back its liveliness and vitality. I noticed an increase in my energy levels, less bloating, and a stable blood sugar level. What made it more rewarding was the realization that I had taken control of my health by making decisions that supported my body's well-being.

In the future, I anticipate a shift in trends toward personalized nutrition that takes into account individual sensitivities and needs. While lectin-free or lectin-limited diets may not be suitable for everyone, for those who have experienced health issues, exploring this approach could potentially bring about significant positive changes.

High-Lectin Foods to Be Cautious of

Lectins serve as nature's security system for plants. They act as the first line of defense against threats like insects, fungi, and micro-organisms. These unique protein molecules attach themselves to carbohydrates on the cell membranes of these invaders, effectively thwarting their attacks and protecting the plant. This is a finely tuned mechanism developed over countless generations of evolution, and allows plants to thrive in a world full of threats.

However, not all plants possess the same levels of lectins in their defensive arsenal. Some plants have evolved to have high levels of lectins as part of their defense strategy. For example, castor beans contain a poisonous substance called ricin, a lectin that can be lethal to both humans and animals. Fortunately, we don't usually include this vegetable in our regular diet.

However, there are plants that we commonly consume that do contain lectins, although in smaller amounts. These include legumes, whole grains, and certain nightshade vegetables like tomatoes and potatoes. Although the lectins found in these foods are less potent, they can still have an impact on our health if consumed in large quantities, especially if the food is raw or not fully cooked.

Lastly, there are some plants that we consume that contain lectins where our bodies have adapted over time to neutralize or minimize their effects. A good example of this is bananas, as they contain a lectin called BanLec. Fortunately, our digestive system has evolved to handle this lectin without it causing any harm.

Understanding the levels of lectins in different foods can help us make more informed decisions when it comes to choosing what we eat. This knowledge can guide us toward a more well-rounded approach to nutrition in Glucotopia.

In Search of Balance

Now, I want to clarify that not all lectins are necessarily bad for us. We should not completely eliminate all foods that are rich in lectins from our diet, as many of these foods also provide nutrients that our bodies need. However, as with everything in life, moderation is key. It's about finding a balance where we can still enjoy a variety of foods without overwhelming our bodies.

Some studies suggest that lectins may be associated with inflammation and gut-related issues such as leaky gut syndrome. There's also speculation about their potential contribution to autoimmune disorders and insulin resistance, although researchers are still exploring these findings (Gong et al., 2017). There isn't a one-size-fits-all solution, and some individuals (including myself) have experienced notable benefits by following a diet low in lectins.

In my experience, adopting a lectin-free diet involved being more mindful of the food I ate and opting for alternatives that were gentler on my body. For example, instead of regular wheat bread, I made the switch to bread without grains. I also replaced tomatoes with cherry tomatoes or prepared de-seeded and peeled tomatoes, which contain fewer lectins. Additionally, I substituted regular potatoes with sweet potatoes. Initially, I had concerns about having limited food options, but I was pleasantly surprised to find a wide range of delicious and nutritious alternatives.

The Link Between Cereal Grains, Lectins, and Inflammation

According to a research paper published in *Nutrients* (de Punder & Pruimboom, 2013), there is a possible connection between consuming cereal grains rich in lectins and inflammation. Cereal grains are widely consumed worldwide and are known to have high levels of lectins. Considering their prevalence in our diets is therefore crucial when considering our health.

As noted above, lectins are proteins that can bind to carbohydrates. Within our bodies, they can attach themselves to the cells lining our system, which can disrupt gut function and contribute to increased intestinal permeability, commonly referred to as leaky gut. When the protective barrier of the gut is compromised, harmful substances like bacteria, toxins, and digested food particles may escape into the bloodstream. This can then trigger a response, leading to inflammation throughout the body.

The research paper takes this argument a step further by establishing a connection between lectins and various health problems. Chronic inflammation is well known for its role in contributing to diseases such as heart disease, cancer, autoimmune disorders, and even insulin resistance, which precedes type 2 diabetes. It can also worsen existing metabolic conditions.

The authors of this study emphasize the benefits of modifying our diet to reduce consumption of lectin-rich cereal grains. This approach could help decrease inflammation and lower the associated health risks. Overall, it adds another piece to the puzzle while underscoring the importance of a mindful approach to diet when managing our health, particularly in relation to metabolic disorders like diabetes.

Glucotopia's Revelations About Lectins

The discovery of Dr. Steven Gundry's work (Gundry, 2017) marked a paradigm shift for our valiant hero, Tabius, and the citizens of Glucotopia. Dr. Gundry's book *The Plant Paradox* shed light on the potential harm posed by lectins, highlighting their role in provoking inflammation and their contribution to an array of health issues, including diabetes.

This revelation was akin to unmasking a concealed adversary. The GlucoBits, once thought to be harmless or even beneficial, were now seen in a different light. They were not just simple energy sources; they could also be carriers of those disruptive Lectonians.

Encouraged by this knowledge, many residents of Glucotopia took decisive action. They made changes to their eating habits, carefully avoiding foods that were high in lectins. Their objective was clear; to counter the infiltration of Lectonians and restore balance and harmony to Glucotopia.

Dr. Gundry's findings served as a turning point, shifting the nutritional narrative within the boundaries of Glucotopia. The citizens became more conscious and selective, understanding that their health and wellness depended not merely on *how much* they ate but, more importantly, on *what* they ate. This marked the beginning of a more mindful, informed, and health-focused era in Glucotopia's history.

So, what was the final verdict? The people of Glucotopia found that a personalized approach worked best. Those who experienced improvements continued with a diet low in or free from lectins, while others who didn't notice much difference decided to reintroduce legumes and whole grains into their meals.

Wheat Germ Agglutinin: A Silent Adversary

Meet wheat germ agglutinin (WGA), another member of the lectin family. WGA silently resides in wheat, including its seemingly healthier version, whole wheat. This little compound might not sound like much, but it can pack a punch when it comes to impacting our health. Imagine WGA as a sneaky character hiding among the regular crowds of GlucoBits in wheat and whole wheat. But WGA isn't just a harmless bystander. This protein is capable of causing quite a ruckus in Glucotopia.

Here's how it operates: WGA is sticky—it has an affinity for attaching itself to cell walls including those found in the gut. This can disrupt the cells' ability to absorb nutrients, leading to various digestive issues. Additionally, WGA's adhesive properties allow it to bind to insulin receptors, which enable GlucoBits to enter cells for energy. Consequently, this can create a scenario where the body's cells become less responsive to insulin, resulting in heightened insulin resistance—an alarming concern for Glucotopia.

This cunning protein doesn't stop there. It also plays a role in triggering inflammation within the body, contributing to health problems. Consistently consuming WGA through wheat and whole wheat can thus establish a cycle of inflammation, impaired nutrient absorption, and increased insulin resistance.

Recognizing the nature and impact of WGA is of utmost importance for the inhabitants of Glucotopia. By having this knowledge, individuals can make choices when it comes to their diet, opting for foods that provide nourishment without any unwanted companions like WGA.

The role of WGA goes beyond causing inflammation, nutrient absorption issues, and insulin resistance. It also plays an intricate and indirect part in contributing to the problem of obesity, which was increasingly prevalent in Glucotopia.

When WGA attaches itself to insulin receptors, it disrupts the process of glucose entering cells. As a result, glucose remains in the bloodstream instead of being utilized by cells, leading to elevated blood sugar levels. To compensate for this, the pancreas releases insulin, which other function is to promotes fat storage and ultimately leads to weight gain.

Additionally, the inflammation triggered by WGA affects the lining of the gut, potentially causing leaky gut syndrome. This condition increases inflammation within the body. Chronic inflammation has been associated with weight gain, as the body attempts to defend itself by producing fat cells to store excess glucose and toxins.

Furthermore, the impaired nutrient absorption caused by WGA can lead to deficiencies in various nutrients. Our bodies may perceive these deficiencies as a form of starvation and respond by slowing down metabolism in order to conserve energy. This can make weight loss efforts challenging while also promoting weight gain.

Hence, the seemingly harmless WGA has the ability to indirectly contribute to the rising issue of obesity among the people of Glucotopia by interfering with insulin function, causing inflammation and disrupting nutrient absorption. If Glucotopia's residents reduce their exposure to WGA, they have a chance of decreasing their obesity risk and maintaining a healthy weight.

Let me share an anecdote. My beloved wife is sensitive to gluten, which is notorious as one of the lectin family members. Yes, Gluten is one of the lectin. Even a small amount of wheat in her diet leads to discomfort, bloating, and an overall feeling of being unwell. Her body quickly displays warning signs against this visitor.

On the other hand, I don't have the same immediate reaction when it comes to wheat. My body doesn't raise an alarm as soon as I consume it. However, that doesn't mean I ignore the effects of wheat and its components. My wife and I have made a mindful decision to steer clear of wheat. For her, it's due to a sensitivity she experiences. As for me, it's about preventing the long-term and subtle impacts of WGA. Instead, we consume millet and sorghum, which are lectin free.

The Evolution of Wheat: From Ancient Grains to Modern Hybrids

Modern wheat and its ancestral varieties differ significantly, with changes that have arisen from years of selective breeding and hybridization. These alterations have been driven by the need for crop varieties that can withstand the challenges of contemporary agriculture and meet global food demands. Here are some key differences:

Genetic Composition:
Ancient Wheat: Varieties like einkorn, emmer, and spelt have simpler genetic structures. Einkorn is a diploid wheat, meaning it has two sets of chromosomes.
Modern Wheat: Modern wheat, specifically the common wheat variety known as Triticum aestivum, is hexaploid with six sets of chromosomes. This complexity arose from hybridization events combining different grass species over time.

Gluten Content:
Ancient Wheat: Generally, ancient wheat varieties have a lower gluten content compared to modern wheat and different types of gluten proteins, which some people find easier to digest.
Modern Wheat: It has been bred to have a higher gluten content, which is advantageous for baking (providing elasticity and chewiness to bread), but this has raised concerns about gluten intolerance and potential health effects for some individuals.

Yield:
Ancient Wheat: These varieties often have lower yields compared to modern wheat, which made them less favorable as agriculture intensified and demanded higher productivity.
Modern Wheat: Bred for high yields, modern wheat varieties are shorter (due to the introduction of dwarfing genes), which makes them sturdier and less likely to lodge (fall over) before harvest.

Nutritional Profile:
Ancient Wheat: They are often cited for their potentially higher nutrient levels, including minerals, vitamins, and antioxidants.
Modern Wheat: While still nutritious, some argue that modern breeding practices have focused more on yield rather than nutritional content, possibly leading to a reduction in certain nutrients.

Pesticide and Fertilizer Use:
Ancient Wheat: Grown traditionally, these crops were often less dependent on chemical inputs, partly due to their lower yields and different growth patterns.
Modern Wheat: It is often cultivated in intensive farming systems that rely heavily on chemical fertilizers and pesticides to maintain high yields and control pests.

Tolerance to Environmental Conditions:
Ancient Wheat: These types have evolved over millennia and are often more tolerant of harsh conditions, such as poor soils and drought.
Modern Wheat: While bred for robustness in a variety of climates, they can be less hardy in extreme conditions without agricultural interventions.

The Importance of These Differences is Multifaceted:

Health Implications: There is ongoing debate about the health effects of consuming modern wheat versus ancient grains, particularly concerning digestive health and chronic inflammation.
   Sustainability: Ancient grains are often highlighted as more sustainable options due to their lower requirements for chemical inputs and their adaptability to organic farming systems.
   Culinary Diversity: Ancient grains offer a wider variety of flavors and textures, contributing to culinary diversity and food culture.
   Agricultural Biodiversity: Preserving ancient grains helps maintain genetic diversity in our crops, which is essential for food security and adaptive agriculture in the face of climate change. Now choice is yours, I will prefer einkorn wheat anyday over modern wheat.

My Personal Journey: The Before and After

I have noticed a reduction in inflammation since I eliminated foods rich in lectins from my diet. Before, I used to have episodes of inflammation that made me feel uncomfortable and sluggish. However, ever since I switched to a lectin-free diet, these occurrences have become much less frequent and not as severe.

Additionally, problems like heartburn and acidity, which used to be a part of my daily life, are now nonexistent. Now that I understand what I was missing, I feel confident and happy about myself. Eating in this way has boosted my productivity in life. I can enjoy meals without the fear of experiencing discomfort or pain afterwards. The change has been liberating and has allowed me to re-discover the joy in eating.

One of the remarkable transformations I've noticed since adopting a lectin-free diet is the clarity of mind it has brought. The brain fog that once clouded my thoughts has lifted, leaving behind a heightened level of focus and mental sharpness that had been absent for a time. Tasks that used to feel overwhelming due to my lack of concentration now seem manageable and even enjoyable.

However, perhaps the most unexpected and rewarding outcome of this dietary change is the stability of my mood. I no longer experience the mood swings that previously would leave me emotionally drained. Instead, I have noticed that my mood stays relatively stable, making it easier for me to go about my day without experiencing emotional disturbances.

Dietary Guidelines for a Lectin-Free Life

Foods to Include:

A lectin-free diet promotes the intake of nourishing, low-lectin foods such as:
- Leafy greens like kale, spinach, and lettuce

- Whole grains such as einkorn, sorghum and millet

- Cruciferous vegetables (e.g., broccoli, cauliflower, Brussels sprouts)

- Low-lectin fruits (e.g., berries, cherries, apples)

- Nuts and seeds (e.g., blanched almonds, macadamia nuts, pecans, flaxseeds, sesame seeds)

- Pasture-raised animal products (e.g., grass-fed meat, pasture-raised chicken)

- Wild-caught fish and seafood

- Healthy fats (e.g., avocado, olive oil, coconut oil)

Foods to Avoid:

The diet recommends avoiding or limiting high-lectin foods, such as:
- Legumes (e.g., beans, lentils, peanuts)

- Whole grains (e.g., modern wheat, barley, oats)

- Nightshade vegetables (e.g., tomatoes, potatoes, eggplants)

- Certain fruits (e.g., melons, tropical fruits)

- Dairy products from conventionally raised animals

- Processed and refined foods (e.g., white bread, sugary snacks)

Preparation Methods to Reduce Lectin Content

Traditional cooking methods can significantly decrease the lectin content in foods, making them safer for consumption. These methods include:
- **Soaking:** Soak legumes and grains overnight in water to reduce lectin content.

- **Fermenting:** Fermenting foods, such as cabbage or yogurt, can help break down lectins.

- **Boiling:** Boiling legumes and nightshade vegetables can inactivate a significant portion of the lectins they contain.

The Scientific Basis:

The reasoning behind these guidelines is that by reducing or eliminating foods that are high in lectins and focusing on nutritious low-lectin options, individuals with diabetes may see improvements in managing blood sugar levels, insulin sensitivity, and overall well-being. The diet aims to minimize the inflammation and digestive issues associated with consuming lectins.

The way I see it, we are all in this together, like a big, happy family striving to build a healthier, happier, and joyful life. I've got this goal, this mission, and I would love for you to join me on it. It's all about beating this silent bad guy called inflammation. Now, you might not see this guy, but trust me, he's there—and he's up to no good.

So, what's my dream? Well, it's to banish this inflammation adversary from every corner of our bodies. Let me be clear—it won't happen overnight. It's not as simple as flipping a switch. This is a marathon, not a sprint.

It requires time, perseverance, and commitment to track down inflammation and kick it out. The great news is that we're all in this together. I'm here to support you every step of the way. And let's not forget we have the ability to regain control, improve our health, and get rid of that inflammation. This is a mission worth fighting for, my friend.

Lessons From Our Ancestors: Ancient Wisdom for Modern Well-being

Our ancestors might have been strangers to the conveniences of modern life, but they knew something profound about balance in their diets. Facing their share of dietary adversaries, particularly lectins, they cultivated a repertoire of natural defenses within their meals, which we can learn from even today.

Envision their diet as a finely-tuned army—kiwifruit leading as the valiant captain with its lectin-neutralizing abilities; okra, the versatile lieutenant, creating a protective barrier; and crustaceans with their chitin armor acting as the steadfast protectors. Cranberries, rich in anti-inflammatory agents, moved with the finesse of fleet-footed messengers across this ancient nutritional battlefield.

Yet, they didn't just defend; they also nurtured. Their diet included a robust array of anti-inflammatory fare—berries bursting with polyphenols, nuts packed with healthy fats, and greens teeming with phytonutrients. These weren't just foods; they were natural allies against inflammation, integral to their daily regimen.

Our ancestors' approach was holistic. They paired lectin-containing foods with those rich in lectin-neutralizing and anti-inflammatory properties, creating a delicate, yet powerful equilibrium. This wisdom seems all the more critical today as we navigate a world where our food systems have introduced new variables into the equation.

The advent of pesticides and herbicides, while increasing agricultural yields, has also presented a new set of challenges for our gut health, potentially increasing inflammation within our bodies. These modern concoctions may disrupt our internal ecosystems, tipping the scales away from the balance our ancestors so carefully maintained.

So, here we are, centuries later, armed with their insights yet faced with new foes. It begs the question: How much of your diet is anti-inflammatory? Are you including foods that can counteract the modern-day assaults on our wellbeing?

And let's not forget about our defenses against lectins. What steps are you taking to ensure your lectin defense is strong? Are you employing the natural strategies that have been handed down to us to keep these substances in check?

Our ancestors may not have had science labs or nutritionists, but their intuitive understanding of diet and its impact on health is something we're only beginning to appreciate. Their legacy is not just in the foods they ate, but in the holistic approach they took to eating.

Now, it's our turn to ask ourselves—how do we uphold and adapt their wisdom in our daily lives? How do we navigate a world that has changed so much, yet still face timeless challenges of health and well-being?

By reflecting on our own dietary choices and considering the wisdom of the past, we can strive to recreate that ancient balance, ensuring that we not only survive but thrive in our quest for a healthy, joyous life.

My Turning Point:

I can still vividly recall the days when I embarked on my lectin diet. Having spent half a year investing my time and energy in a lifestyle overhaul, the hour of reckoning was finally upon me. It wasn't merely about what I was consuming; it went beyond that. I said farewell to lectins, banished sugars, and nurtured a newfound relationship with healthy oils. It was no easy task. I held onto belief in this journey and clung onto hope. I disciplined my life with these healthy options, learning and applying my newfound scientific-based knowledge into my daily life. I could sense the transformation happening within me. My energy levels were at their peak and my well-being experienced an unprecedented improvement.

However, inside me there lingered a hint of doubt that perhaps these positive changes were nothing more than a placebo effect. I got my routine blood work done, which included liver function tests, cholesterol level checks, and, most importantly, the highly anticipated HbA1c test, and then waited anxiously for the results.

My A1c was 7.7% and my fasting glucose levels were 12.0mmol/L, which served as a wake-up call for me to make a complete lifestyle change. I therefore eagerly awaited the results of my update. When I finally saw the notification and checked my numbers, I couldn't believe what I read. My fasting glucose levels had dropped to 5.1 mmol/L and my A1c was now at 5.2%! These figures were a testament to the unwavering dedication and disciplined lifestyle that I had adopted. My heart swelled with joy and pride; it's hard to put into words how incredible this accomplishment felt.

This transformation didn't happen overnight or without effort. It took six months of commitment along with continuous learning, unlearning old habits, and embracing new ones. Every moment was worth it. This victory wasn't about overcoming diabetes; it also reinforced my belief in the healing power of nature and the remarkable resilience of the human body. You know what's even more exciting? This was just the beginning.

Initially, my family doctor had expressed skepticism regarding the benefits of a lectin-free diet. However, when the era of COVID-19 began and our consultations shifted to an online platform, she had the opportunity to observe my progress over the span of a year. The transformations in my well-being were dramatic and undeniable.

During one of our sessions, she took a keen interest in the adjustments I had made to my lifestyle and eating habits. With enthusiasm, I shared my journey with her, explaining the foods I had eliminated from my diet and the positive outcomes I had experienced. She diligently documented all the details, showing curiosity about my newfound approach to managing my diabetes.

The concrete proof of my health manifested through various lab tests. For the first time in a decade, my A1C levels remained consistently stable at an impressive 5.2%. My alanine transaminase (ALT) levels, which had typically stayed above 60, significantly dropped to a healthier 32. And perhaps most visibly noticeable was my weight transformation—I successfully went from weighing 90 kilograms (approximately 198 pounds) down to 72 kilograms (approximately 159 pounds).

Interestingly, the enhancement in my well-being also resulted in a reduction in my expenses. I was spending less on medications, therapies, and doctors' appointments, which provided some relief. It clearly indicated that my health was heading in the right direction.

Chapter Eight

Eating for Nourishment

Putting Nutrient Density Before Taste

I n today's fast-paced world, we have been blessed with numerous conveniences that have made our lives easier. Among these, our food choices have particularly benefited. Supermarkets now offer a variety of flavors and cuisines, allowing us to indulge in delicacies from all over the globe without leaving our homes. However, amid this abundance and accessibility, we seem to have lost sight of the purpose of eating: **NOURISHMENT**.

Food holds an integral place in our lives; it sustains us, brings people together during social gatherings, and is deeply intertwined with our cultural identities. In this modern era, we often prioritize the sensory pleasure and convenience associated with food rather than its nutritional value. Supermarkets are filled with tempting packaged meals that promise instant satisfaction and cater to our desire for diverse tastes, while requiring minimal effort in preparation. As a result, many of us find ourselves making choices based on convenience and immediate gratification, without considering that food's primary function is to provide the essential nutrients our bodies need for optimal functioning.

Over time there has been a shift in how we eat compared to previous decades. The convenience offered by packaged foods, the tempting allure of fast-food restaurants, and the persuasive advertising tactics employed by the food industry have resulted in an excessive focus on taste, often disregarding nutritional value. We have begun to prioritize satisfaction for our taste buds at the expense of considering our long-term health needs. This shift has not only affected our physical well-being but also impacted our understanding and appreciation of food's main purpose, which is to nourish our bodies.

Scientific Evidence of Our Dietary Shifts:

Scientific research makes it clear that our shift toward high-energy, low-nutrient foods has significant implications, directly contributing to the rising prevalence of chronic diseases, encompassing obesity, heart disease, and type 2 diabetes (Duffey & Popkin, 2011).

According to the findings, the average calorie density (calories per gram of food) in our diets has significantly increased. This rise can be attributed mainly to consuming high-calorie foods that are often rich in sugar and unhealthy fats but lack essential nutrients. As a result, our daily calorie intake has skyrocketed without providing us with the vital nutrients required for optimal bodily function.

Glucotopians have a craving for nutrient-rich GlucoBits. However, without realizing it, we have ended up consuming energy-rich but nutrient-poor foods instead. This imbalance in our food intake has disrupted the harmony in Glucotopia, causing an increase in obesity, heart disease, type 2 diabetes, and other chronic conditions.

To make matters worse, the problem has been compounded by trends in portion sizes. Studies have shown that portion sizes have significantly increased over time (Young & Nestle, 2002). Combined with the energy content of modern foods, this leads to us consuming more calories than we actually need. Consuming excess calories can result in weight gain and various health problems regardless of the nutritional value of the food consumed.

The authors of this paper also identified that there was a noticeable difference between the actual portion sizes in the market and the standards set by the U.S. Department of Agriculture (USDA) and the FDA. With the exception of sliced bread, all food portions in the market were significantly larger than those set out in the standards. For example, cookies exceeded the USDA standards by 700%, while pasta, muffins, steaks, and bagels surpassed the standards by 480%, 333%, 224%, and 195%, respectively. In the past, many foods were introduced in sizes that were either smaller than or equal to what we have today.

However, present-day sizes for items like fries, hamburgers, and sodas are now two to five times larger than they were in the past.

Moreover, our eating habits have also seen an increase in how frequently we eat. It's not just that we're consuming larger portions; we're also doing so more frequently. This rise in the number of eating occasions provides opportunities to consume calories, ultimately contributing to the excess energy that fuels issues like obesity and other health concerns.

Understanding Nutrient Density:

In this chapter, we delve into the concept of nutrient density and why it should serve as the foundation of our dietary choices. Nutrient density refers to the ratio of beneficial nutrients to the energy content in foods. Foods with high nutrient density provide substantial amounts of vitamins, minerals, and other beneficial substances while containing relatively few calories. They offer us value for our consumption, maximizing our nutrient intake per calorie consumed. By prioritizing nutrient density, we ensure that every bite contributes to our overall well-being by supplying our bodies with the essential elements necessary for functioning optimally, healing efficiently, and thriving.

However, comprehending and implementing the principle of nutrient density in our day-to-day lives requires a strategic approach, due to today's complex food environment. This environment often leans toward promoting foods that are high in taste but low in nutrient density—foods that provide temporary pleasure but offer little nutritional value. These are like using low quality fuel for our cars; it may work temporarily but in the long run it damages the engine.

The shift toward foods that are high in energy but low in nutrients has a significant impact on our overall health and well-being both at an individual level and within society as a whole. The implications go beyond weight gain and obesity; they encompass a range of chronic diseases, highlighting the utmost importance of having nutrient dense diets.

The significance of nutrient density is not mere speculation; there is an abundance of scientific evidence supporting its role in managing chronic diseases and maintaining optimal health. One notable study shed light on some fascinating discoveries (Camps et al., 2016). This research delves into how the energy density and viscosity of food affect emptying—essentially how quickly food leaves the stomach—and feelings of satiety. It shows that foods with high levels of energy but low viscosity (meaning they are calorie dense but lack fiber and other beneficial nutrients) are quickly digested and don't provide a lasting feeling of fullness. This can result in feeling hungry sooner after consuming such foods, which increases the chances of overeating and subsequently gaining weight.

On the other hand, foods that have lower energy density but higher viscosity—in other words, nutrient-rich foods that are high in fiber—take longer to be digested, promoting a sense of fullness. This not helps control hunger but also ensures a gradual release of glucose into the bloodstream, leading to more stable blood sugar levels.

So, what does this mean for Glucotopia? By relying on nutrient-dense GlucoBits as their primary food source, the residents can maintain a steady supply of energy while avoiding drastic spikes and drops in blood sugar levels. Additionally, feeling satisfied for longer periods helps prevent overeating and supports weight management. Therefore, nutrient-rich foods not only nourish Glucotopia but also contribute to maintaining its overall well-being by reducing the risk of health issues like diabetes and obesity.

Navigating the Food Landscape:

As we move forward, we will explore the process of identifying foods that are rich in nutrients and incorporating them into our diet. This will enable us to enhance our well-being and guide Glucotopia toward a state of equilibrium and success.

Equipped with this knowledge, I will share strategies for including nutrient-dense foods in your meals, even in a world that caters predominantly to our taste preferences. I will offer tips and advice to help you navigate through a food landscape focused on flavors, empowering you to make informed dietary decisions and refocus on nourishment.

Furthermore, I want to dispel the misconception that prioritizing nutrition means sacrificing taste. I will demonstrate how nutrient-dense foods can be equally satisfying and flavorful as their less nutritious counterparts. Through providing examples and drawing on my own experiences, my aim is to showcase that embarking on a nutrient-focused diet can be an enjoyable adventure filled with delicious discoveries.

I extend an invitation for you to join me on this journey toward understanding the essence of food. Together, let's redefine our perspective on eating by placing the emphasis on nourishment rather than mere sensory pleasure, allowing us to reclaim vibrant health through providing our bodies with the high-quality fuel they truly deserve.

Welcome to a world where our diet is not solely controlled by preferences and the satisfaction of eating comes not only from the enjoyment it brings, but also from the nourishment it provides.

The Tantalizing Taste Versus Nutrient Showdown:

Let's take a moment to compare two types of food: a donut and a spinach salad. Which one do you think offers the most nutrients? At first glance, the donut may seem more tempting with its sweet icing and soft texture. However, when we delve into the content of each food, the story changes significantly.

Despite its taste, the donut mainly consists of refined carbohydrates, unhealthy fats, and loads of calories. On the other hand, while the humble spinach salad might not be as appealing to those with a sweet tooth, it is packed with valuable nutrients. It contains vitamins A, C, and K, B vitamins, dietary fiber, calcium, iron, and protein—all while being lower in calories. As a result, the nutrient density of the spinach salad clearly surpasses that of the donut. It provides a range of beneficial nutrients that support overall cell health in Glucotopia, while the donut mainly contributes empty calories and leads to sugar spikes and crashes.

Recognizing this difference marks a step toward shifting our focus from taste alone to nutrient density. This change in perspective doesn't mean sacrificing taste; rather, it encourages finding a balance between delicious flavors and nutritional value.

It's not about eating purely for pleasure; it's about finding a balance between satisfying your taste buds and providing your body with the necessary nutrients. The goal is to transform the act of eating into a holistic experience that benefits both your taste buds and your overall health. Each meal, each bite presents an opportunity to nourish your body and move closer toward an optimum state of health.

Packing for the Journey to Health:

Imagine that every meal or snack is like preparing for a demanding journey—a journey toward better health. You want to pack in as many valuable items (or nutrients) as possible without exceeding your calorie limit. In this analogy, nutrient-dense foods are the essential tools you need for the journey—they are compact yet offer significant value.

Think of nutrient-dense foods as versatile gadgets with multiple functions. They are small, lightweight, and easy to pack, and can serve various purposes—much like how a Swiss Army Knife can serve as a knife, a screwdriver, a bottle opener, and more. On the other hand, nutrient-poor foods are comparable to filling your suitcase with sand. While they may take up space, they don't provide any value or utility for your journey.

When it comes to meals, it's important to think of them as suitcases. A spinach salad may seem simple, but it's actually packed with essential nutrients like vitamin K for blood clotting, vitamin A for vision, iron for red blood cell production, fiber for digestion, and antioxidants to fight harmful free radicals. The best part is, it doesn't come with a high calorie count.

On the other hand, if we opt for a meal full of processed foods like a cheeseburger with fries, we may be consuming a lot of calories but not getting the nutrition our bodies need. It's like carrying around that suitcase filled with sand—heavy on our system but lacking the tools for optimal health.

So, let's make informed choices as we embark on our journey toward Glucotopia. Let's pack our suitcases with nutrient-dense foods that nourish us and give us energy along the way. Of course, taste is important too, but it shouldn't be the sole factor in how we pack our suitcases. Nutrition should always take precedence.

It's worth noting that foods high in nutrient density are often low in energy density. Take carrots and candy bars as an example; one is packed with vitamins and minerals while being low in calories compared to the other. Both the carrot and the candy bar are approximately the same size, but there is a significant difference in their nutritional value. The carrot, packed with vitamins, minerals, and fiber, has a lower calorie content compared to the candy bar, which is high in sugars and unhealthy fats.

The Glucotopia Analogy:

Now let's imagine a truckload of food called GlucoBits arriving in Glucotopia. In one scenario, the truck is loaded with nutrient-rich foods that have low energy density, such as fruits, vegetables, and whole grains. These foods fill up the storage spaces in Glucotopia (your stomach), providing resources for the city's activities without causing overcrowding. The residents of Glucotopia work efficiently, benefiting from having an abundant supply of essential tools and materials to maintain harmony within the city.

In another scenario, the truck arrives at Glucotopia's gates carrying a different type of cargo: Palatabits. These Palatabits are high-energy-density foods, like fried items, sugary drinks, and processed snacks. At first glance, these Palatabits might seem tempting and alluring with their delicious flavors. However, it's important not to be deceived by their appearance.

Once the cargo has been unloaded, the Glucotopians quickly realize that, despite occupying the storage space, these Palatabits don't contribute much to the functioning of the city. They fill up the storage areas rapidly, taking up space but providing very few of the necessary tools and materials needed for efficient operations.

Consequently, the Glucotopians start facing difficulties. The scarcity of resources combined with the crowdedness caused by the Palatabits makes their work more challenging. They become slower, their productivity decreases, and the functioning of the city is disrupted. Harmony gives way to chaos and Glucotopia feels the effects.

This situation beautifully highlights why it's crucial to choose foods that are rich in nutrients rather than simply high in calories. The pleasure of taste is momentary; its impact on our health lasts much longer. So, whenever you're about to eat, remember: you're not just nourishing yourself; you're also nourishing Glucotopia. The quality of that nourishment matters greatly. Make healthy choices by opting for nutrient-dense foods instead of Palatabits and your body—your very own Glucotopia—will express its gratitude.

Prioritizing nutrient density over energy density enables us to fulfill our body's nutritional needs without consuming excess calories. By understanding the concept of nutrient density and incorporating it into our dietary decision-making process, we can ensure that our bodies receive the high-quality fuel they deserve; we should all prioritize nothing less for our bodies.

Nutrient-Rich Food and Diabetes:

Nutrient-rich foods play a role in managing diabetes. Opting for foods with a low glycemic load, a high fiber content, and plenty of antioxidants can help regulate blood sugar levels and reduce the chances of complications related to diabetes. Prioritizing these nutrient-dense options over processed sugary alternatives is an effective strategy in managing diabetes.

The advantages of nutrient-dense foods are extensive, and they have a positive impact on various aspects of our well-being. They bolster our immune system, improve our mood, optimize cognitive function, and promote good gut health, among numerous other benefits. Choosing nutrient-dense foods is like choosing vitality, longevity, and overall wellness.

Embracing nutrient-rich foods over less beneficial options may pose challenges due to the modern food environment we live in today. However, as we'll explore next, embarking on this journey is not only possible but also incredibly fulfilling in numerous ways. The vibrant cities of Glucotopia and Gutville eagerly await the impact of our well-informed decisions. Let's persist in constructing these cities by harnessing the power of nutrient-rich foods.

The narrative shared in the section above titled "The Glucotopia Analogy" strikingly mirrors our real-world predicament. Food companies employ teams of scientists to create what they call "foods." These are foods that really stimulate our senses and make us want to eat more than necessary, which can lead to overeating and weight gain. A study published in the journal *Obesity* looks into this topic in detail (Fazzino et al., 2019).

These hyperpalatable foods are usually high in calories and low in nutrients. They give us a boost of energy, but they don't provide the essential vitamins, minerals, and fiber our bodies need. Over time, relying too much on these kinds of foods can result in nutrient deficiencies and health issues, even if we're consuming enough calories.

Below is how you can ensure you prioritize nutrient-dense foods as part of your diabetes management:

Emphasize Whole Foods:

One of the changes made by the inhabitants of Glucotopia was to prioritize the consumption of whole foods. These are foods that undergo minimal processing and retain their natural state as much as possible. Whole foods possess richness in nutrients and encompass items such as fruits, vegetables, lean proteins, healthy fats, and whole grains. The Glucotopians replaced their PalataBits with fruits and vegetables, lean proteins, and whole grains, thereby providing their city with a plethora of essential nutrients.

Read and Understand Nutrition Labels

The residents of Glucotopia acquired the skill of comprehending and interpreting nutrition labels effectively. This enabled them to spot PalataBits that were cleverly disguised within products. They learned to look beyond the marketing claims displayed on the packaging, and instead focus on assessing ingredient lists and nutrient facts panels in order to make well informed choices. One guideline they followed was that if a food contained an extensive list of ingredients that were difficult to pronounce or recognize, it was highly likely a PalataBit.

Meal Planning and Preparation

To avoid falling back into their old routines, the people of Glucotopia embraced the practice of planning and preparing their meals in advance. They would carefully plan their meals, focusing on including a wide array of nutritious foods. Additionally, they dedicated time to cooking their own meals and snacks, reducing their reliance on packaged PalataBits.

Mindful Eating

Another important habit adopted by the citizens of Glucotopia was mindful eating. The Glucotopians learned to eat without distractions and truly appreciate their food, relishing the flavors and textures of their nourishing meals. By practicing mindful eating, they not only found greater enjoyment in their meals but also developed a better understanding of their hunger and fullness cues, which prevented overeating.

As we wrap up this chapter, it's also exciting to share with you that I'm currently developing a smartphone application specifically designed to assist you during this transition. This app will serve as your own "PalataBit detector," helping you identify and navigate through the hidden realm of PalataBits present in your food choices. By harnessing the power of this technology, you'll be empowered to make decisions about what you eat right from your phone.

Just like in the world of Glucotopia, where advanced technology supported the transition from PalataBits to nutrient-rich GlucoBits, this application aims to assist you in your real-life journey. It will provide you with nutritional information, identify hidden sugars and unhealthy fats, and suggest healthier alternatives. Its purpose is not just to help you understand what you're consuming but also to empower you in making better choices for each meal.

I truly understand that each person's path toward a healthier lifestyle is unique, and personalized guidance can make a significant impact. That's why I'm committed to ensuring that, as soon as this application is ready, it reaches the hands of those who are eager to prioritize nutrient density in their diet.

If you're interested in being among the first users of this application, visit the following link:

www.glutop.com

I will then be able to keep you updated on the app's progress and ensure that you are notified as soon as the application becomes available for download.

Furthermore, apart from receiving updates about the app itself, you will also receive tips, resources, and articles that will support your journey toward prioritizing nutrient density. In this manner, even prior to the app being fully prepared, you will possess the necessary tools and information to begin opting for more nutritious food choices.

I am eagerly anticipating your participation in this new phase of our pursuit toward improved health and wellness. Bear in mind that each stride you take toward consuming nutrient-rich foods is a step closer to a joyous and healthier version of yourself. Together, let us transition from giving importance to taste alone to giving priority to nourishment.

Chapter Nine

The Power of Fermented Foods

Unleashing Gut Warriors

Throughout the course of history, cultures from all over the world have acknowledged and harnessed the power of fermentation—an age-old culinary tradition with significant implications for our health and wellness.

From a scientific perspective, fermentation is like an enchanting microscopic dance of life. It involves a symphony of bacteria and yeast that break down sugars in food into simpler components through a process called enzymatic action. This fascinating process primarily occurs in environments lacking oxygen, known as anaerobic conditions. It's the enchantment that gives us many beloved foods and beverages: the tangy yogurt we enjoy at breakfast, the crispy sauerkraut on our favorite sandwich, the delightful fizz in a glass of kombucha, and the intricate flavors found in a slice of sourdough bread.

Our ancestors stumbled upon this transformative process thousands of years ago. However, it wasn't just about creating new flavors or preserving food. While they may not have comprehended its intricacies back then, they instinctively knew something fundamental: these fermented foods made them feel better, healthier, and more vibrant.

What they were experiencing was the impact that fermented foods had on their bodies, especially when it came to gut health—an aspect we now recognize as crucial for overall well-being. The fermentation process supports the growth of bacteria known as probiotics. Consuming these nutrient-rich foods is akin to sending an army of helpful micro-organisms to your gut—they work tirelessly to maintain a balanced gut flora, aid in digestion, and strengthen your immune system.

The role played by these micro-organisms is twofold. Firstly, they serve as biochemical factories that produce various substances that enhance the nutritional value of food. These substances include vitamins, antioxidants, and other bioactive compounds that have effects on our health. For instance, when milk is fermented to create yogurt, the bacteria *Lactobacillus bulgaricus* and *Streptococcus thermophilus* produce vitamin B$_{12}$, which is crucial for nerve function and the production of red blood cells.

Secondly, these micro-organisms are responsible for the flavors, aromas, and textures found in fermented foods. They achieve this by generating compounds such as lactic acid, which lends fermented foods their distinct tangy taste.

Benefits of Fermentation for Your Gut

When we consume fermented foods, we not only nourish ourselves with the food but also introduce beneficial microbes into our gut. These microbes are commonly known as probiotics and aid in maintaining a balance of gut flora.

The gut is often referred to as our "second brain" due to its significant influence on our overall well-being. It houses trillions of microbes collectively known as the gut microbiota. This diverse community of micro-organisms plays a role in various aspects of our health—ranging from digestion and immune function to even impacting our mood.

Consuming fermented foods can be likened to sending reinforcements to bolster the armies of microbes residing in Gutville. These reinforcements fortify Gutville's defenses, which ensures that harmful invaders are effectively kept at bay.

They play a role in efficiently breaking down and absorbing food, making sure that every GlucoBit delivered is used to its full potential. Moreover, they contribute to preserving the integrity of the gut barrier, preventing substances from entering Glucotopia and causing chaos.

As well as influencing our gut microbiota composition, fermented foods also offer additional advantages for maintaining good gut health. Foods that have undergone fermentation are often easier to digest because the fermentation process breaks down tough-to-digest components. This means that individuals with digestive issues can often tolerate these foods, allowing them to obtain essential nutrients without experiencing symptoms.

If we envision our body's state of health as Glucotopia, then Gutville—a metropolis of micro-organisms in our gut—can be considered one of its major cities. The inhabitants of this city—our gut microbiota—play a key role in our overall well-being. To ensure their existence, we must provide them with appropriate nourishment, and this is where fermented foods come into play.

Fermented foods serve as care packages that we send to Gutville. Packed with probiotics, they not only increase the population of this city but also enhance its diversity—a vital aspect, for maintaining a healthy gut ecosystem.

Current Scientific Findings

The field of gut microbiota research has witnessed an explosion of interest over the past decade. Scientists have begun unraveling the ways in which our gut microbes impact our well-being, and the findings have been truly ground-breaking. We now understand that these tiny inhabitants of our gut contribute to various aspects of our health, from facilitating digestion and nutrient absorption to supporting immune function and even influencing our emotional state.

At the core of this research lies the concept of microbiota diversity, which refers to the multitude of micro-organisms present in our gut. Higher diversity is generally associated with better health. A diverse gut microbiota exhibits more resilience and a better capacity to withstand disturbances such as harmful pathogens or sudden shifts in dietary patterns.

In a research article published in the *Journal of Physiological Anthropology*, the authors explored the effects of fermented foods on both gut microbiota and mental well-being (Selhub et al., 2014). The study revealed that consuming fermented foods rich in probiotics can promote a more diverse gut microbiota. This in turn may have impacts on mental health through the gut–brain connection.

In Glucotopia, having an assortment of beneficial microbes within the gut is analogous to possessing a multifaceted defense system. Each type of microbe contributes its abilities to protect Glucotopia against various threats. Some excel at breaking down certain types of food to provide essential nutrients for Glucotopia's inhabitants. Others specialize in producing substances that strengthen Gutville's walls, preventing unwanted substances from entering Glucotopia. Additionally, some are skilled at communicating with our cells to coordinate an effective immune response.

Types of Fermented Foods

Yogurt, kefir, sauerkraut, and kimchi are examples of fermented foods that contain the beneficial microbes discussed above. When we incorporate these foods into our diet, we introduce microbial species into our gut microbiota and enhance its diversity. This can further improve the function and resilience of Gutville.

Among the range of fermented foods, cheese holds a special place as a beloved delicacy. It has been a star on our tables for generations, as both the main attraction and a delightful accompaniment. The process of creating cheese is truly remarkable, involving the transformation of milk through the actions of specific bacteria, yeast, and molds. These micro-organisms work together harmoniously to convert lactose into acid, giving cheese its distinct flavors and transforming it into a treasure trove of probiotics.

Cheese offers more than just the pleasure of its taste. Beneath its surface lie numerous health benefits, especially in aged cheeses. These cheeses are brimming with cultures that can greatly benefit our digestive system. Similar to those found in yogurt, these microscopic warriors play roles beyond our imagination. They assist in optimizing digestion, enhancing absorption, and strengthening our gut's defense mechanisms to safeguard against digestive ailments.

But there's a question to consider: with the wide selection of cheeses available in the market, how do we choose the best ones? Follow the tips below, and bon appetit!

Consider aging: Typically, aged cheeses like cheddar, parmesan, gouda, or feta are packed with probiotics. As they mature, their lactose content decreases, making them easier to digest and increasing the concentration of probiotics. The aging process also enhances their flavors, providing a gourmet experience.

Read the label: Check cheese labels for terms like "raw," "un-pasteurized," or "probiotic-rich." Pasteurization eliminates beneficial bacteria, so opting for raw or unpasteurized versions ensures you're getting those valuable probiotics.

Prioritize quality: Not all cheeses are made equal. Give preference to traditionally made cheeses rather than mass-produced ones. Local cheesemakers often employ time-honored techniques and allow natural fermentation, which can enhance the cheese's health properties.

Moderation is crucial: While cheese is nutritious, it's also calorie dense and can be high in sodium. It's important to consume it and enjoy it as a special treat rather than an everyday indulgence.

Embrace exploration: The world of cheese offers an array of options. Feel free to experiment with different types of cheese, but remember to prioritize quality and the health benefits it provides over just the taste.

When selected thoughtfully, cheese can offer a culinary adventure while also promoting good health. By understanding the process of fermentation and making informed decisions, we can enjoy every bite knowing that it satisfies our taste buds and contributes to our well-being.

Cheese: The Fermented Powerhouse of Diversity and Flavor:

In the world of fermented foods, cheese stands out as a culinary chameleon. With origins tracing back millennia, cheese is a testament to the ingenuity of our ancestors in preserving milk. Each cheese variety offers a unique combination of textures, flavors, and a host of beneficial microbes that have potential health benefits.

Cheese is the result of milk meeting beneficial bacteria, enzymes, or molds, and this interaction creates a spectrum of fermented products enjoyed across cultures. Not only does cheese enrich our diets with high-quality proteins and essential nutrients like calcium and phosphorus, but certain types also contribute live cultures that can support gut health. Here's a selection of cheeses that can be stars in your probiotic lineup:

- **Cottage Cheese:** A soft, fresh cheese known for its high protein content and lower fat content. It's a versatile ingredient that can be a probiotic-rich addition to meals if it contains live cultures.

- **Ricotta:** This creamy cheese, made from whey, is often fresher than other cheeses and can offer probiotics depending on the preparation method.

- **Cheddar:** This widely loved, aged cheese not only packs a flavorful punch but also comes with the added benefit of beneficial bacteria.

- **Gouda:** A cheese that's not just delightful in taste but also a valuable source of probiotics, making it an excellent choice for those looking to add more fermented foods to their diet.

- **Parmesan and Swiss Cheeses:** These hard, aged cheeses are dense in nutrients and rich in probiotics, making them both delicious and beneficial.

- **Feta:** A brined cheese traditionally made from sheep's or goat's milk, feta contains a variety of microorganisms that promote a healthier gut environment.

- **Blue Cheese:** Its distinctive veins of mold are not just for flavor—they also harbor beneficial bacteria that can withstand the journey through the stomach to the intestines.

When incorporating these cheeses into your diet, moderation is key due to their fat and sodium content. Additionally, look for cheeses that state they contain "live and active cultures" to ensure you're getting the probiotic benefits.

While some cheeses can be enjoyed fresh, the aged varieties are particularly noted for their probiotic content. Aging allows the development of a complex ecosystem within the cheese, where beneficial bacteria thrive. This process not only enhances the flavor but also the potential health benefits.

Identifying Healthful Cheeses in a Sea of Options:

Choosing the right type of cheese is crucial for reaping its potential benefits while minimizing any adverse health effects. To differentiate between healthful and less healthful cheeses, consider the following factors:

- **Quality of Milk:** The best cheeses are made from high-quality milk—ideally, organic and sourced from grass-fed animals. This milk tends to have a better nutritional profile, including higher levels of omega-3 fatty acids and conjugated linoleic acid (CLA), which are linked to anti-inflammatory properties and may aid in weight management.

- **Processing:** Look for cheeses that have undergone minimal processing. Highly processed cheeses often contain added preservatives, artificial colors, and flavors that can negate the benefits of the natural fermentation process.

- **Age:** Aged cheeses typically contain less lactose and are richer in probiotics. Their aging process allows for the development of a complex flavor profile and a breakdown of milk proteins, which some individuals find easier to digest.

- **Fat Content:** While cheese is a source of saturated fats, opting for varieties with a balanced fat content can help manage calorie intake. That said, full-fat cheeses can be part of a healthy diet if eaten in moderation and can be more satisfying, potentially aiding in portion control.

- **Sodium Content:** Some cheeses are high in sodium, which can contribute to high blood pressure and other health issues if consumed in large quantities. Cheeses with lower sodium content are generally a healthier choice.

The European Cheese Advantage

European cheeses often have a reputation for being superior, and there are a few reasons for this:

- **Strict Regulations:** Many European cheeses are protected by Designation of Origin status, which mandates traditional production methods and geographic sourcing. This can lead to a higher quality product.

- **Traditional Methods:** European cheese makers often use raw milk and traditional fermentation methods, which can preserve the cheese's natural probiotics and enzymes.

- **Variety and Biodiversity:** Europe's long history of cheese-making has resulted in a vast array of cheeses, each with its own unique bacterial cultures, which may contribute to a more diverse gut microbiota.

Current and Emerging Research:

Research into the effects of fermented foods on diabetes management suggests potential benefits, particularly in terms of improving glycemic control and insulin sensitivity, though findings are still being explored for definitive conclusions.

A meta-analysis conducted on the intake of fermented dairy foods and diabetes mellitus (DM) risk, which included 15 studies with 485,992 participants, found a statistically significant decrease in diabetes risk with higher intake of such foods. Specifically, higher yogurt consumption was notably associated with decreased DM risk, suggesting a dose-dependent relationship between fermented dairy food intake and lower DM risk. (Zhang et al., 2021)

As the science advances, it becomes increasingly clear that the role of fermented foods goes beyond simple nutrition. They represent a holistic approach to health—a symbiotic alliance with micro-organisms that have co-evolved with humans for millennia, offering their metabolic capabilities in exchange for a place within the thriving metropolis of Gutville.

As we look to the past for wisdom, the age-old tradition of fermentation emerges as a beacon of hope, a potential path to not just manage but possibly reverse the tide of diabetes. It's an invitation to transform our diets and our health, using the tools nature has provided to restore the once prosperous land of Glucotopia to its former vitality.

Incorporating Fermented Foods Into Your Diet

So, how can you incorporate these gut-boosting foods into your meals? Here are a few suggestions:

- **Start small:** If you're new to fermented foods, it's best to begin with small servings. This gives your gut time to adjust. For instance, having a spoonful of sauerkraut as a side dish or enjoying a glass of kefir in the morning can be a great way to begin.

- **Embrace variety:** Experiment with different types of fermented foods. Each one contains specific strains of beneficial microbes that contribute to a diverse gut microbiota.

- **Make it a habit:** Strive to include fermented foods in your meals. It could be as simple as having yogurt for breakfast, sipping on kombucha in the afternoon, or adding some kimchi to your dinner.

- **Try DIY:** Fermenting foods at home can be a fulfilling process. It also allows you to have control over the ingredients and can be cost-effective, too.

- **Get creative with cooking:** Incorporating fermented foods into your dishes can add a new flavor profile. For example, try adding kimchi to fried rice or blending yogurt into smoothies and dips.

Remember, introducing fermented foods into your diet should be a culinary journey rather than a chore. Listen to your body. Go at your own pace. Over time you'll discover your preferred foods and learn the best ways to incorporate them into your meals.

In our journey towards gut health these foods rich in probiotics are like trusted companions. They help nourish our gut microbiota strengthen our body's defenses and support well-being. So why wait? Let's embark on this adventure and unlock the potential of fermented foods for a healthy gut!

Making Your Own Fermented Foods

The world of home fermentation can be both exciting and rewarding. It not only offers a delightful hobby, but also provides numerous health benefits while giving you control over the quality of the ingredients. Additionally, fermenting food at home is a cost-effective way to regularly include these nutrient powerhouses in your diet.

Here are some simple recipes and techniques to kick-start your DIY fermentation journey:

Sauerkraut

To create this fermented food, all you need is cabbage and salt. Start by slicing the cabbage and sprinkling it with salt. Gently massage the cabbage until it releases its juices, then pack it tightly into a jar, ensuring it is fully submerged in its brine. Cover the jar with a cloth or fitted lid to allow the gases to escape during fermentation.

To achieve your desired taste, leave it at room temperature away from direct sunlight for a few days or a couple of weeks.

Pickles

For fermented pickles, gather cucumbers, dill, garlic, and pickling spices. Pack all these ingredients into a jar. Fill it with brine made from saltwater, then loosely cover the jar. Let it sit at room temperature for approximately one week.

Kombucha

If you want to make kombucha, you'll need sweetened green tea and a symbiotic culture of bacteria and yeast (SCOBY), which you can purchase online or obtain from another fermentation enthusiast. Put the SCOBY in the tea, cover the jar with a cloth, and allow it to ferment at room temperature for around one or two weeks. Once it reaches your desired level of tanginess, enjoy it as is. Add fruit or juice for a secondary fermentation to create unique flavors.

Remember that maintaining safety is crucial during home fermentation. Always use clean equipment and fresh, high-quality ingredients. If you notice any signs of mold, or if the ferment has a smell or taste, it's best to discard it for safety reasons. With experience, you'll learn to recognize signs of fermentation such as its sour smell, slight effervescence, and tangy taste.

Embarking on your home fermentation adventure may seem a bit intimidating at first. However, once you take the plunge, it becomes truly captivating to witness the metamorphosis of basic ingredients into intricate, flavorful, and nourishing foods. With some practice and patience, you'll become an expert fermenter, enriching Gutville's landscape with a supply of homemade foods packed with beneficial probiotics!

As we reach the end of our exploration into the realm of fermentation, we can truly appreciate the power these extraordinary foods possess. They are not merely a food category or a passing dietary trend. They serve as a testament to nature's force: tiny microbes that have a profound impact on our health despite their size. They connect us to our heritage, representing a tradition that has been handed down through generations and has stood the test of time.

Chapter Ten

Intermittent Fasting

The Rhythm of Health

I f you recall the story of Glucotopia and their never-ending feast, you'll remember how it led to an unhappy and exhausted Insulina, which ultimately resulted in a dark era of insulin resistance. The Glucotopians' excessive indulgence and lack of rest caused chaos and imbalance. Now picture a different scenario—one where the feast was combined with periods of rest, providing a break for both Insulina and the cellular community. That, my friends, is the concept behind intermittent fasting.

If Glucotopia had an opposite realm, it would be the realm of intermittent fasting: Fastopia. a place where ironically power lay in absence rather than abundance. Here, the streets were not lined with sugar-coated delights; rather, they thrived on a structure and routine that allowed the body to rest, repair, and rejuvenate. This may appear to be an unwelcoming world at first glance, but, in reality, it is quite the opposite. In this realm of Fastopia, I discovered the ability to reverse my unintentional journey that had lasted for years.

Let's envision our bodies as high-performance race cars always prepared to zoom down the track at speed. Every skilled race car driver understands that a car cannot run indefinitely without breaks. Even in high-speed racing, pit stops are crucial for the car to rest, refuel, and undergo the necessary maintenance to ensure optimal performance throughout the race.

These pit stops play a key role because, without them, the car would likely break down or its performance would significantly decline. Similarly, our bodies also require pit stops, which is where intermittent fasting comes into play. Just as a race car cannot constantly operate at high speed 24/7, our digestive system also needs time off from its task of digestion. This break allows our bodies to repair cells, eliminate waste, and restore balance, essentially performing the maintenance required to keep us in good condition.

Intermittent fasting provides our body with this needed rest period. During the fasting window, we refrain from supplying our body with fuel (food) that it needs to process. This shift allows our body to switch gears from digestion mode to restoration and repair mode.

It's important to note that intermittent fasting is not a diet; rather, it's an eating pattern that focuses on *when* we eat rather than *what* we eat. It's a simple concept: dividing your day or week into designated times for eating and fasting. During the eating period you consume your meals, while during the fasting period you refrain from eating. However, the impact it has on our bodies, including on insulin sensitivity, is truly remarkable.

Scientific Evidence for the Benefits of Intermittent Fasting

As we delve deeper into the world of fasting, let's start by exploring the scientific foundation behind this practice. In recent years, fasting has received significant attention from the scientific community, resulting in numerous studies that shed light on its potential benefits.

At its core, intermittent fasting revolves around the principles of energy balance and metabolic regulation. When we eat, our bodies convert food into energy in the form of glucose, which gets stored in the liver. Once our liver reaches its storage capacity for glucose, any excess glucose is converted into fat and stored throughout our bodies. However, when we fast, this process is reversed as our bodies start utilizing fat for energy instead—leading to weight loss.

There are theories explaining why intermittent fasting may improve health outcomes. One notable theory centers around autophagy—a process whereby cells "cleanse" themselves by breaking down and recycling cellular components. This process plays a role in maintaining the overall health and functioning of our cells, and it is believed to be even more beneficial during periods when we abstain from eating.

Furthermore, fasting is thought to have an impact on insulin sensitivity, which can be particularly advantageous for individuals who have type 2 diabetes. When we consume food, our blood sugar levels increase, prompting our pancreas to release insulin. Insulin enables our cells to absorb glucose and utilize it as energy. However, in people with insulin resistance, the cells become less responsive to insulin, resulting in raised blood sugar levels. Research indicates that intermittent fasting has the potential to enhance insulin sensitivity and assist in regulating blood sugar levels (Albosta & Bakke, 2021).

It's like when a cleaning crew comes into Glucotopia after the lights are turned off for the night. The process of "cleaning up"—known as autophagy—helps cells get rid of contaminated proteins and damaged components, which in turn reduces inflammation and potentially slows down the aging process.

Intermittent Fasting and Diabetes

One significant advantage of fasting for individuals with diabetes is its potential to enhance insulin sensitivity. A research paper published in *Cureus* (Lingappa & Mayrovitz, 2022) emphasizes the complex connection between sirtuin proteins (SIRTs) and their potential impact on age-related diseases, particularly diabetes. SIRTs, often referred to as "longevity proteins," play a crucial role in extending lifespan and regulating various biological functions. These proteins act as defenders within our cells, shielding them against the challenges that come with aging.

This study highlights how intermittent fasting can increase SIRT levels, leading to a range of health benefits. Just as the taking of regular breaks via intermittent fasting revitalizes our energy, it also seems to rejuvenate the cellular environment. The higher levels of SIRTs resulting from fasting not only provide protection against age-related decline but also offer resilience against diabetic challenges.

Furthermore, the analysis uncovered promising connections between the use of diabetic medications and SIRTs, suggesting a possible synergistic relationship in managing the disease. Similar to a tuned orchestra producing harmonious music, elevated levels of SIRTs combined with diabetes medications appear to create a more balanced metabolic symphony that could potentially delay complications.

To sum up, when we comprehend and utilize the capabilities of SIRTs and possibly merge them with methods like intermittent fasting, we can establish a strong defense against diabetes and the challenges related to aging. This research suggests the beginning of a more resilient biological domain.

By adopting fasting, we not only provide short-term benefits to our bodies, but also make a substantial investment in our long-term health. It allows our bodies to reset, enhances insulin sensitivity, and effectively manages energy reserves for a happier Glucotopia.

Intermittent fasting serves as a button for Glucotopia, granting the city a chance to take a break, re-evaluate its resources, and promote more efficient management. This pause often makes all the difference between chaos and harmony within the city, showcasing the potential of fasting in managing type 2 diabetes.

Additionally, intermittent fasting can support weight management—a further aspect of type 2 diabetes control. As mentioned earlier, it influences energy balance and contributes to weight loss while reducing central obesity, which is closely linked with insulin resistance.

Another intriguing advantage of fasting lies in its potential to alleviate inflammation, a prevalent issue among individuals with diabetes and a factor contributing to insulin resistance. A pilot study published in the *World Journal of Diabetes* highlights that intermittent fasting can effectively reduce inflammatory markers, thereby promoting better overall health (Arnason et al., 2017).

Inflammatory markers, also known as cytokines, act as messengers, facilitating cell communication during immune responses. In a functioning Glucotopia, these markers are vital and beneficial for combating invaders or injuries. However, excessive production of these markers can trigger a state of heightened awareness, contributing to chronic inflammation and subsequent health complications.

This study sheds light on one aspect of intermittent fasting: its influence on inflammatory markers. It suggests that intermittent fasting has the ability to regulate communication activity by lowering the levels of inflammatory cytokines in the body. This reduction in inflammation holds advantages for the residents of Glucotopia by promoting improved overall health.

The reduced inflammation allows Glucotopia's defenses to relax a bit, focus on maintenance tasks, and become more efficient when real threats occur. With decreased inflammation, the body also becomes better at managing glucose levels, significantly lowering the risk of developing complications associated with diabetes like heart disease, kidney problems, and nerve damage.

This study highlights the benefits of intermittent fasting. Apart from its effects on weight management and insulin sensitivity, it also supports the immune function and inflammatory response in the body, promoting balance and overall well-being in Glucotopia. It demonstrates how strategic dietary patterns can influence our body's communication networks to contribute to improved health.

Mitochondria and the Benefits of Intermittent Fasting

In the grand scheme of Glucotopia's operations, the city's power plants, which are known as mitochondria, play a crucial role. These powerhouses are responsible for generating the energy needed to support all activities, making them essential for Glucotopia's prosperity.

Similar to bustling cities that never sleep in our world, Glucotopia operates around the clock. Its mitochondria tirelessly work to produce the energy required for every function within this lively metropolis. Their primary task is to convert glucose and fat into usable energy, just like dedicated factory workers who transform raw materials into valuable commodities.

However, there is a consideration to bear in mind: even the most industrious factories require periodic maintenance and re-calibration. This principle applies to our bodies as well. Continuously supplying fuel to our bodies—or, in our analogy, constantly providing a stream of GlucoBits to Glucotopia—can strain our mitochondria.

When our mitochondria are incessantly bombarded with fuel, their efficiency may decline over time. They may struggle to keep up with the influx of GlucoBits and produce energy at a slower rate. Additionally, this continuous energy production process can lead to an increase in compounds called reactive oxygen species (ROS), which have the potential to cause damage at a cellular level. We can call it the "pollution" caused by the internal overcombustion.

Furthermore, a research study published in *The International Journal of Biochemistry & Cell Biology* presents another piece of evidence (Vidali et al., 2015). This study not only supports the impact of intermittent fasting on mitochondrial function, but also emphasizes the beneficial role of specific dietary approaches such as the ketogenic diet.

Intermittent fasting and the ketogenic diet share common ground. Both lead to a metabolic state where the body switches to burning fat for energy instead of carbohydrates. This metabolic state, known as ketosis, triggers physiological changes, one of which is the improvement of mitochondrial function.

During ketosis, when the body utilizes fat for fuel, it produces molecules called ketones. Some of these ketones, like beta hydroxybutyrate (BHB), not only serve as fuel but also act as potent signaling molecules. BHB has been discovered to activate genes for mitochondrial biogenesis, effectively stimulating the creation of new mitochondria and enhancing existing ones.

Imagine if Glucotopia's power plants suddenly not only had improved functioning but also multiplied in number. The outcome would be a city capable of efficiently managing the influx of Gluco-Bits. The study by Vidali et al. provides evidence supporting the idea of intermittent fasting as a beneficial strategy for managing diabetes and improving overall health. However, it is important to approach shifts like the ketogenic diet with caution, taking into consideration individual health needs and preferably seeking professional guidance.

In summary, intermittent fasting shows promise in managing diabetes, enhancing overall health by directly impacting cellular energy production. By adopting this practice, we are supporting our bodies at a fundamental level, ensuring the optimal functioning of Glucotopia and its neighboring regions.

Let's take the example of our eyes. The retina, which plays a role in our vision, has one of the highest concentrations of mitochondria in our body. This is because converting light into information requires significant energy, hence the need for abundant cellular powerhouses.

However, with great power comes great responsibility. Because our eyes contain a number of mitochondria, they are more vulnerable to damage caused by the ROS that I mentioned earlier as "pollution." This oxidative stress can harm eye cells and potentially contribute to eye-related disorders such as age-related macular degeneration and diabetic retinopathy. Eyesight issues may be related to the mitochondria putting in so much overtime work.

Like the rest of our body, our eyes require rest and proper care. By incorporating practices such as maintaining a healthy diet, limiting excessive screen time, wearing sunglasses to shield against UV rays, and overall leading a healthy lifestyle, we can promote the well-being of our eyes. Additionally, taking breaks through fasting can aid in the repair and optimal functioning of the mitochondria not only in our eyes but throughout our entire body.

It is essential to give our mitochondria breaks to allow them to cleanse, repair, and prevent excessive production of harmful elements. By doing we support cellular health and reduce the risk of various health concerns.

Incorporating Intermittent Fasting Into Your Life

Incorporating intermittent fasting into my lifestyle wasn't about skipping meals or depriving myself. It was about re-evaluating Glucotopia's established eating patterns to offering my body a much-needed break. It allowed the gatekeepers of Glucotopia—insulin—an opportunity to rest and reset, leading them to become more efficient in managing GlucoBits.

I started with short periods of fasting and gradually increased them as my body adjusted. On some days I followed a 16:8 fasting routine (16 hours of fasting and 8 hours where I could eat), while on other days I opted for a 12-hour fast.

Getting used to this lifestyle change in Glucotopia was quite a challenge. The streets that were once constantly bustling with activity now had moments of peaceful serenity. There was a rhythm to it all—an ebb and flow that the city had to adapt to. As time went on, something remarkable began to occur: the Glucotopia that used to be consumed by its need for fuel started finding balance and tranquility in these pauses.

Resisting the temptation to indulge in every tempting GlucoBit that crossed my path wasn't easy. However, the feeling of empowerment that accompanied my decision to wait and allow my body to utilize its stored energy was truly liberating. I started to feel less controlled by my meal and more attuned to the actual needs of my body.

The constant feelings of hunger gradually subsided, to be replaced by a clarity and a steady supply of energy.

By adjusting the timing of my meals, I experienced a transformative shift. I could shift my focus away from eating toward nourishing and healing. As a result, not did my Glucotopia survive, it thrived.

Keep in mind that embarking on this journey doesn't require perfection. It involves taking small, consistent steps toward better health. So, grant your body—your very own Glucotopia—the gift of intermittent fasting. Let it find its rhythm and its equilibrium, and witness as it undergoes a remarkable transformation, revealing a healthier and more resilient version of itself ready to face any challenge. It's a journey worth embarking on.

Always remember that each one of us is unique, just like every city has its distinctiveness. Consequently, the fasting routine that suits you best may differ from what works for others. Consult with your health-care provider and listen to your body—honor its signals. And keep in mind that intermittent fasting isn't about depriving yourself; it's about giving your body (your Glucotopia) the time it needs to rest, heal, and revitalize.

So, here's to reshaping our relationship with food and timing—allowing our internal city (like Glucotopia) to thrive in harmony. Let's celebrate the potential of intermittent fasting!

When Should You Eat?

Now let's shift our focus to a key aspect of intermittent fasting: deciding when to eat, and the exact time frame during which you will allow yourself to consume food and experience the influx of GlucoBits into Glucotopia.

An important thing to remember about fasting is that it's not a one-size-fits-all approach. It's essential to align your eating window with your lifestyle and daily routine. The timing of your fasting should complement rather than complicate your life. This will ensure that you can sustain your fasting routine in the long run, where the true benefits of this practice come into play.

Consider your daily rhythms and energy levels. If you're someone who naturally wakes up early and starts their day with vigor as soon as dawn breaks, an earlier eating window might be ideal for you. This way, you can fuel yourself with breakfast and lunch while abstaining from food during the evening and night when you're winding down.

On the other hand, if you tend to be more active during the evenings and prefer staying up late, a later eating window could work better for you. This means skipping breakfast but having your designated time for consuming food perhaps from noon until 8 p.m. This approach can prove beneficial if your social or family activities often revolve around dinner time.

Keep in mind that there are no rules when it comes to intermittent fasting. The key is to find a way that works for you, where it is effective, sustainable, and beneficial for your health. Listen to your body, pay attention to your energy levels and hunger cues, and select an eating window that feels natural and manageable for you.

Intermittent fasting isn't about punishing your body by depriving it of food; instead, it's about establishing an eating schedule that promote good health, energy, and overall well-being. So, let's make good choices on this journey towards a thriving Glucotopia.

The Importance of Discipline

If there is one force that quietly yet powerfully propels success in any endeavor, it is discipline. It is an underestimated but incredibly influential virtue that can ignite profound change when fully embraced. You might question how discipline relates to managing your health or specifically practicing fasting—well, the answer is, discipline is *everything*.

Consider an example from nature that perfectly illustrates the essence of discipline—the universe. Take a moment to reflect on it. Every day without fail, the Sun rises in the east and sets in the west. This remarkable phenomenon has been happening for billions of years, playing a role in maintaining the seamless functioning of our world. The consistency and discipline exhibited by the Sun are what sustain life on our planet. If this order were to falter slightly, our existence and the balance of life as we know it could be at risk.

Now, let's explore how this concept applies to us and our pursuit of health and well-being. Like the unwavering path followed by the Sun, we too need to establish and commit ourselves to a consistent routine when incorporating strategies like intermittent fasting into our lives.

The success of fasting relies heavily on maintaining precise timing and staying dedicated, adhering strictly to the designated eating and fasting periods.

Think of discipline as a muscle that grows stronger with use. Consider an athlete preparing for the Olympics, following a routine, sticking to their diet and workout plan, and making —all in the name of discipline. They embody discipline not only on good days but also during times when motivation is low.

Likewise, when we embark on a journey of fasting or any health regimen, it's perfectly fine to stumble along the way. The key lies in getting up, maintaining that sense of discipline, and persevering.

Discipline goes beyond being a habit; it becomes a way of life. It involves choosing between immediate desires and long-term aspirations. It means focusing your mind on a goal and staying committed to it. It's about making changes today that your future self will be grateful for. After all, achieving better health and wellness is not a sprint but rather a marathon—one that demands consistency, resilience, and, above all else, discipline.

Understanding and Navigating Hunger During Fasting

Fasting can be a way to practice discipline and self-control while giving our bodies a break from the constant work of digestion. However, it can sometimes be difficult to interpret the signals our bodies send during fasting. Whether you're new to fasting or trying to improve your fasting routine, these straightforward tips can offer guidance throughout the process:

Start Gradually

If you're new to fasting, begin with a shorter fasting period and gradually increase it over time. For example, start with a 12-hour fast. Extend the fasting period by an hour each week until you reach a comfortable fasting window.

Stay Hydrated

During fasting periods, it's important to stay hydrated by drinking water. This helps curb hunger pangs and prevents dehydration.

Ah yes, we are now venturing into a new territory within the human body! It's interesting how sometimes our body's communication system can get a bit confused. This leads to a situation where we mistake signals of thirst for signals of hunger.

Yes, you got it right. There are times when our body tells us it needs hydration. We misunderstand it and think it's asking for food! Now you might be wondering, how does this mix up occur?

Well, the way our body reacts to dehydration can be quite similar to how we react when we need to eat. We might feel a drop in energy levels, have trouble focusing, or even hear our stomach rumbling—all of which can easily be misinterpreted as hunger pangs. Remember these could also be signs that our body is desperately asking for a refreshing drink of water.

So, next time you feel like having a snack, take a moment to pause. Before grabbing something to eat, try quenching your thirst first. A glass of water or a cup of tea might just do the trick in satisfying the supposed hunger. By doing so, not only will you keep yourself well hydrated, but you will also avoid unnecessary snacking and the resulting intake of extra calories.

This simple tip can prove to be incredibly useful in managing your diet and maintaining balance in your body—ultimately leading to improved health. Let's keep in mind that satisfying our hunger is not the goal here. It's equally important to understand what our bodies truly need and respond appropriately. So, here's to being more mindful of staying hydrated and reducing snacking!

Tune Into Your Body

Each person may have a different response to intermittent fasting. It's crucial to listen to your body and make adjustments to your fasting routine if necessary. If you experience weakness, dizziness, or any discomfort, you might want to consider shortening your fasting period or seeking advice from a health-care professional.

Make Good Food Choices When You Break Your Fast

When breaking your fast, focus on consuming nutrient-rich foods. This will help replenish your body's stores and support overall health.

Remember to be patient as you embark on intermittent fasting. It may take some time before you start noticing the benefits. Be kind to yourself and remember that this is not a race; rather, it's about making changes in the long run.

Incorporating physical activity alongside intermittent fasting can further enhance its advantages. However, ensure that you time your workouts around your eating window so that you have energy for exercise.

To make your intermittent fasting journey more manageable, consider using a fasting app. These apps can assist you in tracking your fasting and eating windows, monitoring your progress, and offering tips and resources along the way.

As we conclude this enlightening exploration into fasting, let's take a moment to appreciate the irony that sometimes "less is more". By intentionally scheduling periods where no GlucoBits (or any food) is consumed, we empower the guardians of Glucotopia, encourage energy management, and enhance the well-being and vitality of all of the residents in our city.

Chapter Eleven

Exercise and Physical Activity in Diabetes Management

The Power of Movement

There's something I haven't mentioned yet about the citizens of Glucotopia: they tended to be quite sedentary. They seemed to have forgotten the joy of movement, opting to just sit around and wait for the next round of GlucoBits, and only rarely engaging in physical activities. This lack of motion—a contrast to their earlier vibrancy—resulted in a slow-paced way of life. Their contentment and reluctance to change significantly contributed to the era of insulin resistance, which cast a long shadow over the city's future.

What if things had been different? Let's take a moment and journey to Movella, Glucotopia's cousin, where things truly diverge. Unlike the residents of Glucotopia, who had grown accustomed to sitting for long periods of time, the people of Movella were always on the go. The city thrived with an energy and vitality that was impossible to ignore.

From sunrise till sunset, Movella's inhabitants were active and bustling. They didn't push themselves excessively, participate in daily marathons, or perform weightlifting sessions every moment of the day. They weren't slaves to a fitness routine; instead, they had mastered a balanced and sustainable lifestyle.

Their daily routines were filled with a variety of activities—some walked, some danced, some lifted weights, and others stretched their muscles. The key was that they kept moving. This continuous motion wasn't seen as a chore but rather as a part of their lives. They walked to the marketplace, took the stairs, enjoyed gardening, and danced in the evenings, each activity showcasing their dedication to staying active.

This active way of life energized Movella's inhabitants, ensuring optimum functioning of its cells and well-maintained gates guarded by the diligent Insulina. The transport of GlucoBits flowed smoothly and seamlessly, like a perfectly coordinated dance. As a result, the citizens enjoyed health and happiness while avoiding the grasp of insulin resistance—all thanks to their consistent movement and the equilibrium it brought.

Similar to how Glucotopia warns us about the dangers of leading a sedentary lifestyle alongside excessive consumption, Movella proudly stands as a symbol of hope for an active, healthy existence and the numerous benefits it bestows upon our overall well-being. As we delve deeper into this chapter, let Movella serve as a reminder of how crucial it is to incorporate regular physical activity into our lives and how profoundly this can transform our health.

Alright, let's venture away from the sedentary path and explore the vibrant and bustling streets of Movella—a city that thrives on physical activity and growth.

Benefits of Physical Activity for People With Diabetes

The reality is, when you are diagnosed with diabetes, your relationship with your body undergoes a transformation. It's no longer an entity that merely exists—it becomes a landscape that you learn to navigate, a puzzle that you strive to solve, and a city that you aim to govern. In the governance of Glucotopia, exercise plays a vital role.

Think of it as an elixir. It helps lower blood glucose levels, improves insulin sensitivity, aids weight loss, reduces the risk of heart disease, boosts mood, and so much more. Each time you engage in physical activity, it's like fueling the engines of Glucotopia and keeping the city alive and thriving.

The Impact of Physical Activity on the Body

For Glucotopia to operate at its best, maintaining a flow of GlucoBits is crucial. Having too much or too little can cause chaos, with the city's residents either overwhelmed by an excessive amount or struggling due to scarcity. This is another area where physical activity plays a role, as it acts as a regulator of GlucoBits within Glucotopia.

From a physiological perspective, exercise has a significant impact on how our bodies handle glucose. When we engage in activity, our muscles, the bustling factories of Glucotopia, require more energy to function properly. As a result, they utilize the GlucoBits in our bloodstream, effectively reducing blood glucose levels.

To put it simply, think of exercise as a "diplomat" that negotiates the terms for GlucoBits to enter the muscle factories. Regular physical activity makes the factories more receptive, allowing GlucoBits to enter easily and be converted into energy. This process helps maintain levels of circulating GlucoBits in the bloodstream.

What's particularly interesting is that during exercise our muscles become more responsive to insulin. It's almost like Glucotopia's gates are opening wider and allowing GlucoBits to enter efficiently. This increased insulin sensitivity can last for hours or even up to a day or two after exercising, contributing to longer-term control over glucose levels.

What Type of Physical Activity Is Best—And How Much?

Regular exercise is widely recognized as important—and when I say exercise, I mean any type of physical activity. However, in the realm of exercise, there's something known as the "Goldilocks Principle," which is all about finding balance. Not too little, not too much; just the right amount to maintain optimal health and effectively manage conditions like diabetes. This principle holds significance for individuals living with diabetes because both insufficient and excessive exercise can lead to complications. So, what does science tell us about finding that sweet spot in terms of the frequency, intensity, and type of exercise for people with diabetes?

Research indicates that incorporating a combination of exercises along with resistance training is beneficial for managing diabetes (Kirwan et al., 2018). Engaging in aerobic exercise such as walking, cycling, or swimming can have positive effects on cardiovascular well-being and enhance the body's ability to respond to insulin. Meanwhile, resistance training aids in the development of muscle mass, which is vital, for regulating glucose levels.

Another study, published in the *Journal of the American Medical Association*, aimed to understand the impacts of different types of exercise on patients with type 2 diabetes (Church et al., 2010). To conduct the study, the researchers divided the participants into four groups: a control group, an aerobic exercise group, a resistance training group, and a combined exercise group. The aerobic exercise group focused on activities such as treadmill walking, stationary cycling, and elliptical training. The resistance training group primarily used weight machines and free weights. Meanwhile, the combined exercise group participated in both aerobic exercise and resistance training. Each exercise group engaged in their activities three times per week for a period of nine months.

Upon completion of the study, it was observed that both aerobic exercises and resistance training individually proved effective in reducing levels of hemoglobin A1c. However, it was notable that the greatest reduction occurred among those who combined both types of exercises. These findings suggest that taking a combined approach to exercise by incorporating both aerobic activities and resistance training may be highly beneficial for individuals diagnosed with type 2 diabetes.

This is supported by a position statement from the American Diabetes Association (Colberg et al., 2016). This statement presents evidence highlighting the benefits of engaging in both aerobic and resistance training for individuals with type 2 diabetes. It emphasizes that these types of exercise can enhance insulin sensitivity by improving the muscles' ability to utilize GlucoBits, thereby aiding in their management. Additionally, the role of exercise in weight management is emphasized, as this is crucial for controlling diabetes. Regular physical activity, especially when combined with dietary changes, can lead to weight loss and a reduction in fat mass. In our analogy of Glucotopia, this would mean less pressure on the insulin gatekeepers and a more efficiently functioning city.

According to further information from the American Diabetes Association (n.d.), adults with diabetes should aim for least 150 minutes of moderate to vigorous aerobic activity spread out over at least three days each week, with no more than two consecutive days without exercise. They also suggest incorporating resistance training into the exercise routine at least twice a week if their health permits.

However, it's important to remember that these are guidelines and the ideal amount of exercise can vary from person to person based on factors such as age, fitness level, and overall health. This is where personalized exercise planning becomes crucial, as it considers an individual's needs, preferences, and goals.

A further concept to be aware of when thinking about how much exercise to do, and how to fit it into your daily routine, is "exercise snacking"—a kind of snacking that we can all get behind! Research published in *Diabetologia* introduced the idea of reimagining exercise as small bursts of activity, similar to snack-sized portions (Francois et al., 2014). The authors investigated how these short but intense bursts of exercise affected individuals with insulin resistance. They found that this type of "exercise snack" before meals was more effective at controlling blood sugar in people with insulin resistance than a daily 30-minute session of moderate exercise.

So, the next time you feel like having a snack, why not try taking a brisk walk around the neighborhood or doing a quick run up and down the stairs instead? These short but intense bursts of activity might be the secret to keeping Glucotopia functioning at its best!

The Best Time for Physical Activity to Improve Blood Sugar Control

Researchers from the Netherlands explored the best time to exercise for better blood sugar control (van der Velde et al., 2022). The study analyzed data from over 6,000 individuals aged between 45 and 65. The researchers assessed their activity levels and identified when they were most active.

Their findings suggest that engaging in exercise during the afternoon or evening is more effective in managing blood sugar levels compared to spreading activity throughout the day. Morning exercise, on the other hand, did not offer any advantages. Overall, being active during the afternoon or evening was associated with up to a 25%

improvement in blood sugar control compared to being active at other times of the day.

Although the exact reasons why afternoon or evening activity yields better results are still unclear, it appears that our bodies may respond favorably to exercise later in the day. Therefore, if you're aiming for blood sugar control, it might be worth considering scheduling some of your exercise sessions for the afternoon or evening.

All of this leads us to one important conclusion. Exercise in all of its forms is an invaluable tool for managing Glucotopia, by ensuring that there is a regulated distribution of GlucoBits.

My Journey Toward Embracing Exercise

Now, I want to be clear about something: I have a love–hate relationship with exercise. There are days when the mere thought of putting on my sneakers and hitting the road feels like conquering Mount Everest. Then there are those moments where the rush of adrenaline, my racing heartbeat, and the sweat pouring down my face make me feel truly liberated. It's been quite a journey of ups and downs, resistance, and acceptance. It's a journey I'm thrilled to share with you.

Let me assure you that my journey toward embracing exercise wasn't without its challenges. I faced an initial lack of inertia, skepticism, and physical discomforts, and struggled to find time amid my busy schedule. Yet here I am today—more energetic than ever before, while being healthier and having better control over my own Glucotopia. This lifestyle shift didn't require hours at the gym, expensive memberships, or fancy equipment. It all began with something simple: regular walks, an activity I easily incorporated into my daily life.

Over time, I also incorporated resistance and strength training exercises into my routine. My days now have a rhythm, filled with movement and activity just like the lively folks of Movella.

On some days I enjoy a walk in the park or take a refreshing swim in the nearby pool. Other times I find solace in gardening under the warm sun or lose myself in the rhythm of music, dancing freely. The activities may vary, but their essence remains unchanged: I am constantly on the move.

Incorporating Exercise Into Your Routine

Understanding the science behind the importance of exercise is half the battle. The other half lies in putting that knowledge into practice and incorporating activity into our everyday lives, which is precisely what we will address next.

When it comes to establishing an exercise routine, it's crucial to note that diving into a workout regimen overnight isn't necessary. The key lies in starting by setting realistic goals, then gradually increasing the intensity and duration of your workouts as your fitness level improves. An effective exercise routine should ideally include a combination of cardio exercises, resistance training, and flexibility exercises.

If needed, seek guidance—especially if you have underlying health conditions or are new, to certain types of physical activity. Remember that our goal isn't necessarily to become athletes or bodybuilders (unless that's what you desire!). It's about embracing a lifestyle that includes regular physical activity, promoting overall well-being, and, most importantly, finding joy in our lives.

So here's to stepping up, quite literally and metaphorically, to ensure our internal city remains vibrant and dynamic, mirroring the energetic streets of Movella. In the words of the physician Dr. Robert Butler, "If exercise could be packaged into a pill, it would be the most widely prescribed and beneficial medicine in the country" (Ortolan et al., 2022). We all deserve that prescription: a pathway to a more fulfilling life, where we don't just survive but truly thrive!

Here's how you can get started.

Set Achievable Goals

Aim for least 150 minutes of moderate-intensity aerobic activity per week, coupled with strength training on two or more days. Remember, a few minutes of physical activity is better than none. It's crucial to keep in mind that every bit of movement matters. Sometimes we tend to think in terms of "all or nothing," believing that if we can't dedicate an hour to a workout it's not worth doing at all. However, this couldn't be further from the truth. Even brief periods of activity such as taking a leisurely walk around your neighborhood, engaging in a 10-minute strength training session, or doing household chores can accumulate and have a significant positive impact on your overall health.

When setting exercise goals, it's crucial to consider your current fitness level. If you've been inactive for some time, it's best to avoid jumping into intense workouts as they may do more harm than good. Instead, start with low-intensity exercises like walking or gentle yoga. Gradually increase the duration and intensity as your fitness improves. The key is to prioritize consistency rather than focusing solely on intensity. Remember that establishing a routine that you can maintain in the long run is what matters most.

Always keep in mind that the objective isn't to become an athlete; it's about improving your health, managing your blood glucose levels effectively, and enhancing your overall quality of life. Avoid pushing yourself to the point of exhaustion or injury. Seek out activities that bring you joy and anticipation so that exercise becomes not just a routine but also a delightful part of your daily life.

One of the core principles we embrace in Glucotopia is "Progress, not Perfection." It's not about achieving a perfect workout session or attaining an ideal body image. Instead, we focus on making strides toward better health and well-being over time.

Every step you take, every pedal you push, and every movement you make is significant, bringing you closer to a healthier and happier Glucotopia.

Listen to Your Body

Regular exercise should leave you feeling good, not exhausted. If you start feeling tired or encounter any pain, dizziness, or shortness of breath, it's essential to take a break. It's crucial to recognize that your body has its unique rhythm and capacity. It communicates through signs and symptoms, letting you know when it's time to push forward or take a step back. Learning how to listen and respond to these signals can make a difference in your exercise journey.

If excessive fatigue sets in during or after your workout, or if you feel lightheaded or uncomfortable in any way, it's your body signaling that it needs rest. Don't disregard these signs; instead, allow yourself the time for rest and recovery. Overexertion can lead to injuries and burnout, ultimately delaying progress on your fitness journey.

For individuals managing diabetes, monitoring blood glucose levels is of the utmost importance. Physical activity generally helps lower blood glucose levels, which is typically beneficial. However, if glucose levels drop too low, it can lead to a condition called hypoglycemia, or low blood sugar, which can be potentially dangerous. Common symptoms of hypoglycemia include trembling, perspiration, light-headedness, confusion, and, in severe cases, loss of consciousness. To prevent hypoglycemia, it is advisable to check your blood sugar levels after engaging in physical activity. Additionally, keeping a source of fast-acting carbohydrates such as fruit juice or glucose tablets nearby during workouts is a wise precautionary measure.

Incorporate NEAT Activities

Non-exercise activity thermogenesis (NEAT) refers to the energy expended during activities that are not related to sleeping, eating, or exercise similar to sports. These activities encompass tasks like walking to the store or cleaning, as well as small movements like fidgeting. NEAT can vary significantly from person to person, thus playing a role in daily energy expenditure and contributing toward weight management and overall metabolic health.

When it comes to managing diabetes, incorporating more NEAT activities can offer advantages. The continuous but moderate energy expenditure associated with NEAT can enhance insulin sensitivity and contribute to better control of blood glucose levels. One of the things about NEAT is that it doesn't require dedicated time slots like traditional exercise; instead, it seamlessly integrates into our daily lives.

To increase your NEAT, you can make adjustments to your everyday routine. This might include opting for the stairs instead of the elevator, parking your car further away from your workplace or a store entrance, or even moving around while talking on the phone.

By adding more NEAT into your day, you not only burn extra calories but also enhance your metabolic health, which is particularly beneficial for managing diabetes. It underscores the idea that every bit of movement matters and emphasizes that leading an active lifestyle extends beyond just going to the gym.

Staying Motivated

Remember, the purpose of incorporating exercise into your routine is to improve your health and overall quality of life, rather than striving for perfection. Even small changes can have an impact. So, embrace the journey, celebrate every bit of progress you make, and enjoy the process of moving toward a happier Glucotopia!

Embarking on a fitness journey is similar to embarking on any life quest—it requires not only initial motivation but also determination to stay committed. The residents of Glucotopia understand this well, acknowledging the significance of maintaining consistency alongside effort to ensure the prosperity of their city. Here are a couple of strategies to maintain your motivation and dedication to your workout regimen:

Establish SMART Objectives

Make sure your fitness goals are Specific, Measurable, Achievable, Relevant, and Time-bound. SMART objectives offer guidance and facilitate tracking of your progress. Remember, progress regardless of how small it may seem is still progress.

Discover Activities You Enjoy

Physical activity doesn't have to feel like a task. Find activities that bring you joy and anticipation. You can try dancing, cycling, hiking, practicing yoga, or even engaging in gardening. Remember, the most effective exercise is the one you can consistently engage in.

Embrace Variety

Adding diversity to your workout routine not only keeps things interesting but also challenges different muscle groups and enhances your overall fitness.

Establish a Consistent Schedule

Create a workout routine that seamlessly fits into your life. Whether it's a morning yoga session, a midday stroll, or an evening workout, find the time slot that works best for you. The key is to integrate exercise into your lifestyle so that it becomes easier to maintain.

Seek Support

Enlist the company of a workout buddy, join a fitness class, or consider hiring a trainer. Having someone to exercise with can make your workouts more enjoyable and provide an extra layer of motivation and accountability.

Acknowledge Your Victories

Take pride in recognizing and celebrating every achievement along the way, regardless of how small they may seem. Each step forward deserves recognition and celebration.

Practice Patience

Remember that fitness is not a destination but rather an ongoing journey. It takes time for changes and improvements to become visible, so be patient with yourself throughout the process. Keep in mind that the objective is to bring about lasting transformations, not opting for temporary solutions.

Weekly Exercise Schedule for Optimal Blood Sugar Management

Monday
- **Morning**: Short burst of exercise (e.g., 10 minutes of brisk walking or stair climbing)

- **Afternoon/Evening**: 30 minutes of aerobic exercise (e.g., cycling, swimming, or a brisk walk)

Tuesday
- **Morning**: Exercise snack (e.g., 10 minutes of high-intensity interval training)

- **Evening**: Resistance training (e.g., weightlifting session focusing on major muscle groups)

Wednesday
- **Morning**: Exercise snack (e.g., 10-minute brisk walk)

- **Afternoon/Evening**: 30 minutes of aerobic exercise (e.g., jogging or aerobic class)

Thursday
- **Morning**: Short burst of exercise (e.g., 10 minutes of vigorous yard work)

- **Evening**: Resistance training (e.g., bodyweight exercises or using resistance bands)

Friday
- **Morning**: Exercise snack (e.g., quick session of jumping jacks or brisk walking)

- **Afternoon/Evening**: 30 minutes of leisurely activity (e.g., gardening, dancing, or a leisurely bike ride)

Saturday
- **Active Rest Day**: Engage in light activities such as stretching, yoga, or a leisurely walk to stay active without exerting too much strain on the body.

Sunday
- **Morning**: Exercise snack (e.g., a quick circuit of push-ups, squats, and lunges)

- **Afternoon/Evening**: Enjoy a longer session of moderate exercise (e.g., a hike, a long bike ride, or a longer swimming session)

Important Notes:

- **Customization**: This schedule should be adjusted based on individual health status, fitness levels, and medical advice.

- **Consistency**: Aim for at least 150 minutes of moderate to vigorous aerobic activity spread across the week.

- **Resistance Training**: Include at least two sessions per week, focusing on different muscle groups.

- **Timing**: Whenever possible, schedule more strenuous activities or longer sessions during the afternoon or evening for better blood sugar control.

- **Flexibility**: Feel free to swap activities to fit personal preferences and lifestyle.

Some Final Thoughts on Exercise

The ancient Greeks had a saying, "Mens sana in corpore sano," which translates to "a healthy mind in a healthy body." This philosophy encapsulates the essence of exercise. It's not solely about building muscles, shedding weight, or breaking records. It's about cultivating a relationship with oneself, understanding one's limits, and pushing those boundaries. It's about mental resilience, emotional strength, and physical prowess.

Exercise shines bright as a ray of hope. It goes beyond being a routine—it serves as a powerful tool to combat irregularities in blood sugar levels and acts as a protective shield against potential complications.

Let's not underestimate the significance of NEAT either. The small everyday movements we make, like pacing or toe-tapping, subtly but significantly boost our metabolism.

Furthermore, finding the right balance between aerobic exercise and resistance training is crucial. While aerobic exercise enhances our health, resistance training strengthens our muscles. Together they create a symphony of well-being and vitality.

As we wrap up this segment, let's always remember that exercise is a commitment—a promise to take care of both body and mind. Embrace its nature, stay curious, and remain physically active. The journey toward fitness might be long, but it is immensely rewarding. Onward to the exciting adventure!

Chapter Twelve

Elimination of Toxins

The Guardians of Our Health

In the core of Glucotopia, where cells gracefully sway and every-thing appears idyllic, there exists a story whispered in hushed tones but seldom fully comprehended. It revolves around the presence of intruders known as persistent organic pollutants, or POPs for short. These cunning culprits lurk within our surroundings, stealthily infil-trating our bodies and gradually wreaking havoc.

Toxins refer to substances that can cause harm to our bodies. They can originate from various sources, including our environment, diet, and lifestyle choices. Once these toxins enter our bodies, they have the potential to interfere with physiological processes, one of which is the metabolism of glucose.

Amid the spectrum of environmental hazards, a class of conta-minants POPs stands out for their particular tenacity and potential for harm. These chemicals, which encompass by-products, pesticides, and additives found in everyday products, resist breaking down in the environment and remain present for extended periods. What makes them more concerning is their ability to accumulate in living organ-isms' tissues—including humans—through the food chain. This has implications for human health and specifically relates to the develop-ment of type 2 diabetes.

In this chapter, we will explore strategies to minimize our exposure to toxins and enhance our body's natural detoxification processes. We will delve into the idea of restoring the health of Glucotopia, our city, and its inhabitants' well-being one cell at a time. Together. we can tackle this adversary and pave the way toward a life free from diabetes.

Impact of Toxins on Our Health

Our bodies face an attack from various toxins. They enter through the air we breathe, the food, we enjoy, the water we drink, and even seemingly harmless products we use. These hidden adversaries may go unnoticed by our senses and have a profound impact on our well-being.

My understanding of these toxins didn't come from journals or health articles; rather, it began with a conversation. During a chat with a close friend, phthalates came up in discussion and piqued my curiosity. As I delved deeper into the subject, I was astonished to discover that it wasn't just phthalates; numerous other toxins from nonstick Teflon cookware and similar sources were silently finding their way into our bodies.

The conversation with my friend didn't just open my eyes; it led me to explore. As I delved deeper, I discovered the network of toxins that contribute to different health issues, including my own struggle with diabetes. It became clear to me that in order to regain my health and restore balance in Glucotopia, it was crucial for me to confront and understand these intruders.

As we navigate through this chapter, we will unveil these hidden foes, comprehend their workings, and, most importantly, equip ourselves with knowledge to counteract their effects. Together we will learn how to strengthen Glucotopia's defenses and ensure the well-being of its inhabitants—the cells that define our identities.

So, are you prepared to encounter these adversaries and rally the protectors of our health? Let's embark on this journey together.

The Connection Between Toxins and Diabetes

You might be curious about the connection between these trespassers and the realm of diabetes. After delving extensively into the research literature, I stumbled upon an intriguing study titled "Persistent organic pollutants and type 2 diabetes: A critical review of review articles" (Lee et al., 2018). Its promise to unravel the web of links between these pollutants and the onset of diabetes caught my attention.

Here's a summary of what I discovered:

The covert link: Beneath the surface of various studies lies a recurring theme: individuals exposed to higher levels of POPs appear to tiptoe closer to the risk zone for type 2 diabetes. It's almost as if these toxins whisper sinisterly, leading astray the cells residing in Glucotopia. The mechanics of this treachery involve sabotaging insulin pathways, meddling with the energy-producing centers of our cells (the mitochondria), and kindling inflammatory fires.

Not all studies sing the same song: Like any tale, there are variations in the narrative. Some research voices sang louder of the toxin–diabetes link, while others hummed a more cautious tune. Factors like the types of POPs, the level of exposure, and the population studied added their unique notes to the chorus.

Digging deeper: The article didn't simply accept these stories at face value. It delved further by examining other reviews, highlighting potential limitations, and emphasizing how important it is to pay attention to each narrative's subtleties.

A call to action: With concerns about pollutants casting a shadow in various aspects of our world, and diabetes becoming increasingly prevalent, understanding this troubling relationship becomes a matter of utmost importance. There is a call for more researchers to delve deeper into this narrative and unravel its mysteries.

Within Glucotopia's collection of stories, the tale of pollutants and diabetes remains an ongoing journey. This story urges us to pay attention, gain knowledge, and take action, making sure that the smooth coordination of Glucotopia's cells is not disrupted by these intruders.

To further elaborate on POPs, they are enduring compounds that can travel through air, water, and soil to reach remote corners of our planet. The very characteristics that make them valuable in industry and agriculture—stability and solubility in fat—are also what render them hazardous.

These substances have the ability to dissolve in fats easily and are not easily broken down, which leads to their accumulation in the tissues of animals and humans over time. This process is known as bioaccumulation.

POPs enter our bodies through various pathways. They can contaminate crops and be consumed by animals, which then eat, thus entering our food chain. We can also consume them through water or inhale them as part of polluted air. Once inside our bodies, these pollutants can impact our systems by interfering with hormonal signals causing inflammation and disrupting metabolic processes.

Air Pollution

The air we breathe is perhaps the most common source of toxins. Urban environments in particular are notorious for their poor air quality due to vehicle emissions, industrial pollutants, and other particles in the air. Indoor air can also be contaminated with volatile organic compounds (VOCs) released by household products, furniture, and building materials.

Contaminated Water

Our water supply can also be a source of toxins as it may contain harmful substances such as heavy metals, pesticides, pharmaceutical residues, and by-products of water disinfection.

Processed Foods

Processed and packaged foods often contain chemical additives including artificial colors, preservatives, flavor enhancers and sweeteners. These substances can disrupt our metabolism and contribute to insulin resistance.

Personal Care and Household Products

Conventional personal care items like shampoos, lotions, and cosmetics as well as household cleaning products are packed with chemical ingredients that can pose risks to our well-being. These chemicals may include substances known as endocrine-disrupting chemicals (EDCs) such as phthalates and parabens, which have the potential to disrupt hormone function and potentially contribute to metabolic disorders.

Plastic Containers

The use of plastic containers for storing food or drinking water can expose us to harmful chemicals like bisphenol A (BPA), an Endocrine Disrupting Chemical (EDC) that has been linked to various health concerns, including diabetes.

Non-Organic and Processed Meats

Animals raised conventionally are often subjected to hormones and antibiotics that can leave behind residues in the meat we consume. Additionally, processed meats frequently contain preservatives like nitrates and nitrites, which have been associated with health issues.

By understanding these sources of toxins, we can empower ourselves to make informed decisions about the products we choose and the environments we live in. In the following section, we will explore strategies for minimizing exposure to these toxins and promoting a healthier, more balanced lifestyle.

Strategies to Reduce Toxin Exposure

Now that we have an understanding of where toxins can hide in our lives, it's time to take action and minimize their impact on our health. In this section, we will explore strategies that you can implement to significantly reduce your exposure to toxins, lessen their effects, and improve your overall well-being.

The world we live in is filled with sources of harmful substances that can have a negative impact on our health, sometimes without us even realizing it. While some of these sources like pollution are beyond our control, there are many others that we can manage to significantly reduce our exposure to toxins. Making choices like consuming organic, pasture-raised, and wild-caught foods, drinking filtered water, and using natural personal care and household cleaning products can have a meaningful impact on reducing the toxins that accumulate in our bodies.

It's important to remember that every small step toward minimizing toxin exposure matters. You can take significant strides in protecting your health by focusing on eliminating toxins using the following strategies.

Embrace a Healthy Diet

The first step in defending ourselves against toxins is through the food we eat. Choose unprocessed foods that are free from artificial additives and preservatives. Whenever possible, opt for fruits and vegetables that are grown without synthetic pesticides or fertilizers. Likewise, consider selecting pasture-raised meats to avoid exposure to hormones, antibiotics, and other harmful substances.

Switch to Natural Personal Care and Household Products

Replace conventional personal care products and cleaning supplies with natural alternatives. Look for products that contain simple ingredients, or try making your own. There are plenty of do-it-yourself recipes for various items, like hand soap or laundry detergent.

Filter Your Air and Water

To ensure clean air and water and if you can afford it, it's a good idea to invest in a high-quality air purifier that can help reduce indoor air pollutants. Additionally, consider using a water filter to remove potential contaminants from your drinking water. If you're able to, its recommended to have the air and water quality in your home tested so you can better understand the pollutants you may be dealing with.

Limit Use of Plastic

Another important step is to limit your use of plastic, especially when it comes to storing food and water. Opt for glass or stainless-steel containers instead. Avoid heating food in plastic containers as this can cause chemicals to leach into your food.

Support Your Body's Natural Defenses

Incorporating practices that support your body's natural detoxification processes is also beneficial. Regular physical activity helps eliminate toxins through sweat, while maintaining a fiber-rich diet supports gut health and facilitates toxin removal. Including detoxifying foods like vegetables, berries, turmeric, and green tea in your diet can further aid this process.

Go for a Checkup

Don't forget about medical checkups either. These checkups allow you to monitor your exposure to toxins and assess any impact on your health. Certain tests can even detect levels of toxins such as heavy metals in your body. Discuss any concerns with your health-care provider, who can provide guidance on monitoring your health.

Let's keep in mind that it's not realistic to eliminate all sources of toxins in our modern world. However, by making informed choices and adopting healthier practices, you can greatly reduce the amount of toxins your body is exposed to, which can lead to better metabolic health and overall well-being. The power is in your hands. Together, let's create an environment in Glucotopia that supports the well-being of every cell in our city!

Detoxification: The Body's Natural Defense

Our bodies have mechanisms to protect us from harm. They possess systems that are designed to neutralize and eliminate toxins, acting as a natural defense against the harmful substances we encounter daily. These detoxification processes take place in organs like the liver, kidneys, skin, lungs, and gut, each with its own unique role in cleansing our system.

The liver is often referred to as our body's detoxifier. It performs a two-phase process where toxins are broken down and prepared for elimination. In phase one, enzymes are used to convert toxins into less harmful substances. In phase two, these substances become water soluble so they can be eliminated through urine or bile. Any disruption in these processes can result in the buildup of toxins, which can contribute to health problems, including insulin resistance and diabetes.

Our kidneys continuously filter our blood, eliminating waste products and excessive substances, which are then excreted through urine. Sweating helps our skin get rid of toxins and regulates body temperature. Additionally, our lungs expel waste gases from our system.

Furthermore, our gut plays an important role in detoxification. A healthy gut microbiota, with the assistance of fiber, aids in binding toxins and facilitating their elimination through feces. Moreover, specific gut bacteria can directly neutralize certain toxins.

Recognizing these natural detoxification mechanisms highlights the significance of supporting them. So, how can we accomplish this? Here are some lifestyle habits that can enhance your body's detoxification processes:

Stay Adequately Hydrated

Drinking water supports kidney function, aids digestion, and promotes healthy skin, all of which are essential aspects of detoxification. Aim for least 8 cups of water per day, or more if you're physically active or live in a warm climate.

Consume a High-Fiber Diet

Including dietary fiber in your meals promotes gut health, as fiber assists in toxin removal and has the ability to bind to specific toxins, reducing their absorption. Make sure to incorporate plenty of fiber-rich foods into your daily meals. These include fruits, vegetables, whole grains, nuts, and seeds.

Exercise

Engaging in physical activity is beneficial for detoxification in various ways. It improves blood flow, which helps transport toxins to the organs for elimination. Additionally, exercise stimulates sweating, allowing toxins to be expelled through the skin.

Ensure Sufficient Rest

Giving our bodies enough sleep is crucial to allow them to rejuvenate and undergo detoxification processes. It is recommended to aim for 7–9 hours of sleep a night to support these peak detoxification activities.

Moderate Alcohol Intake and Avoid Smoking

Both alcohol consumption and smoking can impede the body's detoxification mechanisms, as well as introduce additional toxins. It is advisable to limit alcohol intake to moderate levels and completely abstain from smoking.

Incorporate Detoxifying Foods into Your Diet

Certain foods are known to promote detoxification processes. For example, vegetables such as broccoli and Brussels sprouts contain a compound called sulforaphane, which can enhance liver detoxification. Additionally, foods rich in antioxidants like berries, green tea, and spices such as turmeric can help neutralize toxic substances and protect cells from damage.

Illuminating Detoxification: The Role of Red and Near-Infrared Light

Beyond the foundational pillars of hydration, nutrition, physical activity, and rest, there exist additional strategies that may bolster our body's detoxification efforts. Among the frontier of wellness innovations is red and near-infrared light therapy—an advanced technique that has gained attention for its potential to support the body's natural detoxification pathways.

This therapy utilizes specific wavelengths of light to penetrate tissues, stimulating cellular energy production and aiding in the repair and rejuvenation of cells. The effects of red and near-infrared light are not superficial; they reach deeply into the body, potentially enhancing blood flow, reducing inflammation, and supporting the liver and skin in their detoxifying roles.

For those who do not have access to specialized light therapy devices, the benefits of red and near-infrared light can still be harnessed through mindful exposure to natural sunlight. The early morning and late afternoon sun provides these beneficial wavelengths, offering a natural and cost-effective method to tap into the detoxifying advantages of light. Incorporating routine outdoor activities during these times can synergize with hydration, diet, and exercise to fortify the body's resilience against toxins.

As we continue to explore the myriad ways to support our health, incorporating varied detoxification strategies, including exposure to red and near-infrared light, can be a valuable part of a holistic approach to well-being. While this area of health technology continues to evolve, what remains clear is the importance of nurturing our body's innate ability to heal and protect itself— a task that is best approached from multiple angles.

By adopting these practices, we can support our body's innate detoxification systems, reduce our toxin load, and improve our overall well-being. As we aid our bodies in eliminating these substances more effectively, we lay the foundation for better glucose metabolism and a healthier future.

Harnessing the Power of Light: Red and Near-Infrared Therapy for Detoxification and Energy Enhancement

In the quest for optimal health, we often overlook a powerful ally that's both ancient and cutting-edge: *LIGHT*. Red and near-infrared light therapy, also known as photobiomodulation, has emerged as a remarkable tool for enhancing detoxification and boosting energy levels.

The science behind this therapy is fascinating. Red and near-infrared wavelengths of light penetrate the skin, reaching deep into tissues, muscles, and even cells. Here, they work their trick, interacting with mitochondria—the powerhouses of our cells—to stimulate the production of adenosine triphosphate (ATP), the energy currency of the cell. This process leads to a cascade of beneficial effects, including:

- Enhanced cellular energy, contributing to better overall vitality and performance.

- Support for the body's natural detoxification processes by increasing blood flow, which helps in transporting nutrients and oxygen to the cells and waste products away.

- Reduction in oxidative stress and inflammation, which are often linked to a variety of chronic diseases, including type 2 diabetes.

For those who can invest in a red and near-infrared light therapy device, the convenience of at-home treatment can make it a valuable component of a daily wellness routine. But for many, such devices may not be within reach financially. However, this doesn't mean the benefits of these healing wavelengths are out of bounds. Here are some strategies to naturally incorporate red and near-infrared light into your life:

Sun Exposure: The simplest way to get red and near-infrared light is from the sun. Early morning or late afternoon sunlight can provide these beneficial wavelengths without the higher risks of UV exposure that midday sun can bring. Aim for 10 to 20 minutes of exposure during these times.

Candlelight: While not as intense as sunlight or therapy devices, the flame from a candle emits a spectrum of light that includes red and near-infrared wavelengths. Engaging in activities by candlelight in the evening can not only provide a calming effect but also offer some level of therapeutic light.

Incandescent Bulbs: Old-fashioned incandescent bulbs are an excellent source of red and near-infrared light. Consider using them in a desk lamp or reading light to receive some therapeutic benefits.

DIY Light Therapy: While not a replacement for more sophisticated equipment, you can create a makeshift light therapy source using red and infrared LED lights available on the market. Ensure safety and consult with experts before attempting to create your own device.

Diet: Certain foods are known to enhance mitochondrial function and complement light therapy. Foods rich in antioxidants, such as leafy greens, berries, nuts, and seeds, can support cellular health and energy production.

Mindful Movement: Gentle exercises, such as yoga or Tai Chi, performed outdoors can provide the dual benefits of physical activity and light exposure, enhancing blood flow and energy levels.

While high-tech devices offer a concentrated form of red and near-infrared light therapy, there are accessible ways to harness the power of light naturally. By integrating these strategies into your life, you can tap into the detoxifying and energizing benefits of light and contribute to the well-being of your cellular city, Glucotopia.

Embracing a Toxin-Free Lifestyle for Improved Health Tomorrow

As we wrap up our exploration of the world of toxins, it becomes evident that chemical exposures are an undeniable aspect of our lives. However, it's important to understand the harm these toxins can cause so that we can make smarter choices and minimize our exposure whenever possible.

It can be overwhelming to navigate through the toxins in our environment. It's important to remember that achieving absolute purity is nearly impossible in today's world. Instead, our goal should be to reduce exposure and support our body's natural detoxification processes.

Every small change we make can make a difference. It might be as simple as choosing organic for the "dirty dozen," opting for a glass water bottle over plastic, or dedicating an extra hour to sleep each night. The "dirty dozen" is a term coined by the Environmental Working Group to describe the 12 fruits and vegetables most commonly contaminated with pesticides. Currently, they are strawberries, spinach, kale, nectarines, apples, grapes, peaches, cherries, pears, tomatoes, celery, and potatoes. Each step, however small it may seem, is a victory in reducing your toxic load and supporting your health.

It's also essential to remember that our bodies are remarkably resilient. When provided with food, water, air, and enough rest, they have the capacity to repair, restore, and rejuvenate themselves. By minimizing toxin exposure and supporting our body's natural detoxification systems, we create the conditions for improved health and well-being.

In your pursuit of a life free from harmful substances, remember that you are not alone. Each one of us has a part to play. By working together, we can bring about a positive transformation toward a healthier and more joyful future. As we minimize the presence of toxins in our lives, we pave the way for a flourishing Glucotopia—a place where our cells, like its citizens, can thrive and prosper.

So, my dear readers, as we embark on this journey together, let us wholeheartedly embrace this toxin-free lifestyle. Rather than viewing it as an arduous or restrictive task, let's see it as an empowering and liberating way of living that promises us a brighter and healthier tomorrow. Here's to a toxin-free, healthier Glucotopia!

Chapter Thirteen

Stress Management and Self-Care

The Calming Power

Welcome to Peaceville, a town nestled within the lively and bustling Glucotopia. However, Peaceville hasn't always been so serene. It used to be just as chaotic and stressful as the rest of the city. Then something changed. The residents of this town came to realize that their constant state of anxiety was actually exacerbating the situation, fueling the growing problem of insulin resistance.

In our world, stress is an all too familiar aspect of our lives. We've all experienced those knots in our stomachs, rapid heartbeats, and sleepless nights caused by worries beyond our control. Science has revealed how stress, much like that prevalent in Glucotopia, can wreak havoc on our bodies and result in a multitude of health issues, including diabetes.

This realization set me on a journey toward self-care and managing stress. I started by making one change in my mindset: I decided not to worry about things that were beyond my control. Whether it was the weather, traffic, people's actions, or even the COVID-19 pandemic, I made a conscious choice not to let them affect my peace of mind.

I began envisioning my life as a lake; external stressors like traffic, the actions of others, or the global pandemic were akin to stones being thrown into this lake. Naturally, they would create ripples and sometimes even waves. However, I came to understand that it was entirely up to me whether I allowed these waves to disturb the tranquility of my lake or if I allowed the water to eventually settle back into calmness.

I made a decision to release things that were beyond my reach and create space for serenity in my life. If I couldn't control the weather, there was no point in fretting over it. When stuck in traffic, instead of letting it unsettle me, I saw it as an opportunity to listen to a podcast or enjoy some music. People's actions were their own choices and I consciously chose not to let them dictate my inner peace.

The global pandemic, while extremely challenging, had aspects that were beyond my control. As a result, I focused on the things I could manage: adhering to safety guidelines, taking care of my health, and offering support to others whenever possible.

This change in perspective was both empowering and transformative. It felt like unburdening myself from a backpack during a hike. I experienced a sense of lightness, harmony with my surroundings, and an improved ability to respond to situations. Similar to the residents of Peaceville, I found myself transitioning from anxiety to proactive tranquility.

How did I attain this state of calm? It required patience, regular practice, and implementing various strategies. I started by practicing mindfulness and meditation and relying on prayer, while also taking responsibility for my actions following the HAPPINESS formula. Additionally, I became more mindful of the moment. To maintain my well-being, I incorporated consistent exercise and followed a balanced diet rich in nutrients. I prioritized getting high-quality sleep each night. Moreover, connecting with loved ones and participating in hobbies and activities that brought me joy played a role.

This method of dealing with stress reflects the wisdom found in a verse from the Bible, which says, "Who of you by worrying can add a single hour to your life?" (Luke 12:25). When we constantly worry about the future or dwell on the past, we lose out on enjoying the moment. It disturbs our peace and can even have negative effects on our physical well-being.

So, come along with me. Step into Peaceville. Let's prioritize self-care, effectively manage our stress levels, and work towards becoming a more balanced and healthier version of ourselves.

Understanding the Role of Cortisol in Stress

When faced with stress, our bodies respond in a way that is both ancient and immediate. The central character in this physiological drama is cortisol, a hormone with a critical role in our fight-or-flight response. Under stress, the adrenal glands release cortisol into the bloodstream, prompting a series of changes designed to temporarily boost our survival capabilities.

Cortisol works by increasing glucose levels in the blood, ensuring that our muscles and brain have enough energy to tackle the immediate threat. This mechanism is vital in short-term, high-stress situations, offering us the burst of energy needed to either confront or flee from danger.

However, the story changes when stress becomes a constant presence. In the ongoing hustle of modern life, where stressors range from work deadlines to personal challenges, cortisol can be chronically elevated. This persistent high level of cortisol has significant implications for our health. It disrupts normal glucose metabolism, leading to sustained high blood sugar levels.

Insulin resistance is a key factor in the development of type 2 diabetes and other metabolic conditions. It illustrates the profound connection between our psychological state and physical health. By understanding the role of cortisol in stress, we can begin to appreciate why managing stress is not just about feeling better mentally but also about safeguarding our physical health.

The Connection Between Stress and Diabetes

The connection between stress and the onset of insulin resistance emphasizes the importance of managing stress effectively—a lesson that Peaceville learned through adversity. By addressing and effectively managing their stress levels, the people of Peaceville could begin transforming their city from a place overwhelmed by stress into a refuge, taking crucial steps toward ending the era of insulin resistance. While this transformation won't be easy, it is necessary for restoring balance in Glucotopia.

The underlying science behind this process is relatively straightforward. When we experience stress, our bodies enter into what's commonly referred to as "fight or flight" mode. This triggers the release of cortisol, adrenaline, and glucagon into our system. This response is crafted to provide a burst of energy—an advantage that our ancestors evolved to have when facing predators or other dangers. The stress hormones prompt the liver to produce glucose, giving our muscles that extra fuel in case we need to fight or flee. At the same time, insulin activity is suppressed to ensure that this additional glucose remains in our bloodstream ready for immediate use.

However, as the world has evolved, so have our sources of stress. We no longer encounter threats like being chased by a lion or going into battle. Instead, our stressors have become less tangible: an overflowing email inbox, seemingly impossible deadlines, unexpected bills putting strain on our monthly budgets, or the challenges of managing multiple roles and responsibilities. Our adrenal glands don't differentiate between a lion and a traffic jam; stress is stress. Consequently, they keep releasing cortisol, which in turn continues flooding Glucotopia with glucose and perpetuates the cycle of insulin resistance.

Although it's impossible to eliminate stress completely, we can definitely control how we respond to it—just like the people of Glucotopia, who made a decision to transform their constant state of heightened alertness into one of tranquility and equilibrium. They came to understand that not every challenge requires a "fight or flight" reaction; sometimes, what we truly need is a "rest and digest" response. This realization brought forth an era in Peaceville where cortisol was no longer an unwelcome guest but rather a hormone that served its purpose and knew when to gracefully step aside. It was this understanding that ultimately restored harmony in Glucotopia.

Strategies to Manage Stress

Understanding the impact of stress on our well-being is crucial. Knowing how to effectively manage it is even more important. Fortunately, there are techniques available that can help tame the stress beast and contribute to a healthier happier life.

It's essential to note that each individual is unique and what may work effectively for one person may not yield the same results for another. Exploring different techniques and discovering the ones that resonate with you and fit into your lifestyle is crucial.

Meditation

One such technique worth exploring is meditation. This ancient practice, which involves focusing one's mind on the moment, has garnered significant attention from the scientific community due to its ability to alleviate stress. A notable study published in 2016 sheds light on its potential benefits, suggesting that mindfulness meditation may not only reduce stress markers but also have positive effects on physical health by reducing inflammation in the body and enhancing immune function (Black & Slavich, 2016).

This holds significance because long-term stress can weaken your body's systems and contribute to various health problems, such as heart disease and diabetes. That's why incorporating mindfulness meditation into your routine can be a good approach to managing stress and improving overall well-being.

Mindfulness meditation involves directing your attention to the moment and accepting it without judgment. It's a practice that has been embraced by cultures worldwide and is now gaining popularity across the world for its potential positive effects on mental and physical health. The beauty of mindfulness meditation lies in its simplicity and accessibility—you don't need any equipment or a specific location, making it accessible to everyone, everywhere.

Integrating mindfulness meditation into your life can be as easy as dedicating a few minutes each day to focus on your breath, pay attention to bodily sensations, or simply observe the world around you. It's about cultivating a sense of presence and tranquility amid our hectic lives. As you continue this practice, you may notice a reduction in stress and anxiety levels while experiencing an increase in feelings of peace and serenity, ultimately enhancing your quality of life.

It's important to keep in mind that mindfulness, like any skill, requires practice. So be patient with yourself throughout this journey.

Over time, you might discover that engaging in this practice not only aids in reducing stress but also improves your ability to concentrate, heightens self-awareness, and deepens your appreciation for the simple moments in life. As a result, it can lead to a series of changes in your overall well-being and health, including better management of glucose levels, which is crucial for residents residing in Glucotopia.

So, why not give mindfulness meditation a chance? It could be the key to attaining a serene and healthier existence within Glucotopia.

Breathing Exercises

Another simple yet powerful tool for managing stress are deep breathing exercises. When we experience stress, our breathing often becomes shallow and rapid. By slowing down our breathes, we can activate the body's relaxation response. The"4–7–8" breathing technique popularized by Dr. Andrew Weil is a good method to begin with. It involves inhaling for four counts, holding the breath for seven counts, and exhaling for eight counts. This technique can be practiced at any time, anywhere, whenever you sense stress creeping into your life.

Self-Care

Amid the pursuit of stress management and optimal health, one fundamental aspect often gets overlooked: self-care. Self-care involves tending to our emotional and mental well-being through activities that nourish and rejuvenate both our body and our mind. It's not a luxury but rather a necessity for maintaining health and effectively managing conditions like diabetes.

Taking care of yourself starts with nourishing your body through nutrient-rich foods. A balanced diet that includes plenty of fruits, vegetables, whole grains, proteins, and healthy fats provides your body with the essential nutrients it needs to function at its best. It's also important to eat mindfully while ensuring you stay hydrated. These habits contribute to your overall nutritional well-being. They not only help manage blood glucose levels but also support sustained energy levels and promote overall health.

Equally important is getting quality sleep. Quality sleep plays a role in various bodily functions, such as glucose metabolism, cognitive function, mood regulation, and immune response. In fact, lack of sleep can negatively impact blood glucose control and insulin sensitivity. That's why establishing sleep habits and addressing any sleep-related issues are crucial aspects of self-care.

Physical activity is another component of self-care. Engaging in exercise improves insulin sensitivity, helps manage blood glucose levels effectively, supports cardiovascular health, and boosts mood. Remember that physical activity doesn't necessarily mean hitting the gym or running a marathon. It can be any activity that gets you moving and brings you joy.

Last—but certainly not least important—is emotional and mental self-care. Building and maintaining social connections, practicing stress management techniques like mindfulness meditation, and engaging in activities that bring you joy are vital for your mental well-being. This is because chronic stress and negative emotions can disrupt the balance of hormones that regulate blood glucose.

Taking care of yourself also involves paying attention to the signals your body sends, taking breaks when needed, and seeking assistance when necessary. It's important to remember that self-care isn't about striving for perfection but rather about consistently making choices that promote your well-being.

Ultimately, self-care acts as a tool on your journey toward improved health and a thriving life. It entails allocating time to nurture both your body and your mind while acknowledging your value. So, go ahead—indulge in a bath, lose yourself in a good book, take a refreshing walk outdoors, or savor a nourishing meal. Here's to prioritizing our well-being so we can lead fulfilling lives!

My Own Journey Toward Peaceville

I used to be someone who constantly pushed myself, handling numerous responsibilities simultaneously while trying to meet exceedingly high expectations. A constant worry about the future consumed me.

This constant state of stress left me feeling exhausted, worried, and out of sync with my body. What's more, it was negatively affecting my blood sugar levels, pushing me deeper into the never-ending cycle of insulin resistance.

Realizing the harm it was causing, I knew I had to make a change. Breaking old habits is not easy and the road to finding inner peace is filled with obstacles. It required a shift in my mindset, moving from trying to control everything to accepting that there are things beyond my control. I had to learn how to let go and find solace in uncertainty, which turned out to be one of the biggest challenges.

To tackle this, I started exploring techniques for managing stress. I began with meditation. At first, my mind would wander relentlessly. Achieving a state of mindfulness felt impossible. However, through patience and practice, I gradually started experiencing moments of calmness and clarity. I learned how to stay present by focusing on my breath and, over time, those moments of tranquility became longer and more frequent.

At the same time, I delved deeper into self-care practices. Prioritizing balanced and nutritious meals became essential for me, along with better eating habits and regular physical activity. Improving my sleep routine also became crucial while ensuring that I stayed connected with my loved ones.

Over the course of time, these practices gradually became a part of my daily routine—not just something I felt obligated to do, but something I genuinely looked forward to.

The changes I experienced were remarkable. I started feeling more connected with both my body and my mind. My blood sugar levels stabilized, leaving me with a heightened sense of energy and vitality. The constant anxiety was replaced by acceptance and a proactive approach to facing life's hurdles. It felt as though I had transitioned from survival to truly thriving.

Of course, there are still things in my life that cause stress. It's a natural part of life. However, the way I perceive and deal with these stressors has changed significantly. Instead of responding with worry and anxiety, I've learned to approach them with acceptance, resilience, and proactive steps.

Sharing this aspect of my journey isn't about portraying a life without stress. It's about emphasizing that change is possible and that embarking on the path of managing stress and practicing self-care is worthwhile. It's about illustrating that the journey itself, with its ups and downs, has the power to transform us into healthier versions of ourselves. In my case, it helped me navigate through tough times in Glucotopia and guide it toward stability and prosperity.

The truth is, stressors will always be present in our lives. They are as much a part of being human as experiencing joy, sadness, or excitement. However, how we perceive these stressors—and, importantly, how we respond to them—can truly make all the difference.

It's easy to view stress as an adversary that needs to be battled or eliminated. What if we were able to shift our perspective and see it as a signal or an invitation to prioritize self-care? Each moment of stress presents an opportunity for self-awareness and personal growth—a chance to connect with ourselves both mentally and physically, reassess what truly matters to us, and nurture our well-being.

Embarking on the journey toward managing stress and practicing self-care might seem overwhelming, especially if you're just starting out. However, remember that even the smallest steps matter greatly. Begin with one change—perhaps engaging in a 5-minute meditation session or taking a short evening stroll.

Chapter Fourteen

The Frugal Gourmet's Guide

Savvy Savings for Glucotopians

I n Glucotopia, the value of food goes beyond its price tag. Instead, it is evaluated based on its nutrient density—the vitamins, minerals, fiber, and other beneficial substances it provides. In our world, there is a belief that nutritious food always comes at a high cost, which often acts as a significant obstacle for many who wish to embark on a journey toward better health. However, this notion is far from reality.

Now, let's address the misconception that has long hindered us from making good choices when it comes to food—the idea that eating well requires substantial financial resources and is only accessible to the wealthy. This misconception has discouraged individuals from even attempting to adopt healthier eating habits. Does healthy eating truly have such exclusivity? Is enjoying a diet high in nutrients something reserved only for the privileged citizens of Glucotopia?

Allow me to share with you what I have learned through personal experience: eating healthily does not necessarily mean breaking the bank. While it's true that certain healthy foods can be expensive, this doesn't mean that maintaining a healthy diet is always cost prohibitive. With some planning, smart shopping strategies, and clever cooking techniques, it's entirely possible to nourish Glucotopia while staying within budget.

I still remember a time when I used to believe that trying to reverse diabetes would cost me a fortune. However, as I went deeper into my journey, I realized that my preconceived notions were holding me back. I discovered that it's not only possible but also enjoyable to eat healthfully on a tight budget. I found excitement in discovering affordable ingredients, satisfaction in preparing meals that were both good for my body and wallet friendly, and the joy of knowing that I could prioritize my health without breaking the bank.

In this chapter, I'll share the strategies and secrets that helped me overcome my misconception about healthy eating. We'll explore everything from planning and budgeting to shopping, and from the art of cooking on a budget to minimizing food waste. Together we can embark on this journey toward nutritious eating.

Planning and Budgeting

Planning and budgeting are crucial when it comes to maintaining a healthy diet on a limited budget. Think of it as constructing a house—you wouldn't begin without a blueprint, right? The same principle applies to your eating habits.

It's important to have a plan in place to avoid making bad purchases and unhealthy food choices and incurring unnecessary expenses. Here are the steps to create your blueprint for healthy eating:

Start with Meal Planning

Before heading to the grocery store, take some time each week to plan your meals. Keep it simple by outlining what you intend to eat for each meal and snack. Take into account the nutrients you need, available cooking time, and your personal taste preferences. Having a meal plan not only ensures a well-balanced diet but also helps you identify exactly which groceries you need, preventing any unnecessary spending.

Prepare a Grocery Shopping List

Based on your meal plan, make a shopping list. This list acts as your defense against impulse purchases and assists in sticking to both your plan and budget. As you jot down the items you need, consider their cost and where you can find them at the best possible price. Additionally, keep an eye out for produce as it tends to be cheaper and fresher.

Set a Food Budget

Determine how money you can realistically allocate toward food expenses on a weekly or monthly basis. Take into account factors such as income and other financial obligations.

Remember, the objective isn't to minimize your food expenses but to maximize the nutritional value you get for your money. Stay within your budget as much as possible but remain open to flexibility. If you come across a great deal on a nutrient-rich food, it might be worthwhile to spend a little extra.

Keep Track of Your Spending

Just like how you monitor your blood glucose levels, keep a close eye on your food expenditures. This will help you understand where your money is going, whether you're adhering to your budget, and areas where you can potentially save. You might be pleasantly surprised to discover that eating healthily can actually be more affordable than anticipated!

Just remember what a blueprint is: it is a guide rather than a rulebook. Your meal plan, shopping list, and budget should be flexible and able to adapt to your changing needs and circumstances. The main goal is to provide Glucotopia with the nutrients it needs without worrying much about the cost. So, lets grab our blueprints and get started!

Smart Shopping: Maximizing Nutrition on a Budget

The grocery store holds a treasure trove of foods. Navigating its aisles can sometimes feel like solving a maze. However, with a few strategies, you can discover gems: affordable yet nutrient-packed foods that will help feed Glucotopia without breaking the bank. Here's your guide to shopping.

Understanding Unit Prices

Unit pricing can be your secret weapon when cost shopping. It lets you know how much a product costs per unit of measurement (such as per ounce or per gram). Typically, you'll find this information listed on the shelf tag below the product. By comparing unit prices, you can determine which brand or size offers the best value for money.

Seasonal and Locally Sourced Produce

Buying fruits and vegetables when they're in season can make all the difference to your budget. Seasonal produce tends to be readily available and less expensive.

In addition, the flavor and nutritional value of seasonal and locally produced food are often, at their peak. It's also worth considering the support of farmers and markets, as they offer grown produce that can be more affordable due to shorter travel distances from farm to market.

Buy in Bulk

When it comes to nonperishable items, think about purchasing in larger quantities. Buying in bulk typically offers a lower price per unit compared to smaller-packaged alternatives. Just make sure you have storage space and that the food won't spoil before you have a chance to use it. There was a great deal on coconut milk in our local Costco. The price in other stores was $3.50/can, but in Costco it was almost $1.50/can. It was a pack of 6 cans and I bought a few of them with ample expiry left. Now, the same pack is $15/pack. I also purchased a good amount of almond flour and monkfruit/erythritol sweetener, and saved so much money in the longer run.

Consider Store Brands

Don't underestimate the value of store brands. They are often less expensive than name-brand products and provide the same quality and nutritional content. Take a look at the ingredients list and nutrition facts to ensure you're not compromising on nutrition for cost savings.

Keep an Eye Out for Bargains

Keep an eye out for sales and discounts but remember to exercise discernment. Just because an item is on sale doesn't automatically mean it's the best choice for your health or budget. Use sales as an opportunity to stock up on nonperishable items or try new nutritious foods that you might not otherwise consider purchasing.

Minimize Waste

Lastly, remember that wasted food can be very costly. Plan your meals ahead of time, store food properly, and get creative with leftovers in order to minimize waste and save money.

With these strategies, you'll be well prepared to navigate the maze of the grocery store and discover the treasure hidden within: a cart filled with affordable foods that will fuel Glucotopia. Enjoy your shopping!

Tips for Minimizing Food Waste

While we're discussing how to feed Glucotopia on a budget, we must consider the impact of food waste. Every bit of food we discard is like throwing away GlucoBits, not to mention the strain it puts on our finances and the environment. So, how can we decrease food waste? Let's delve into some suggestions.

Embrace Your Leftovers

Leftovers can be a lifesaver for both your budget and your time. Don't just see them as meals; get creative! Yesterday's grilled chicken could transform into today's chicken salad. The stir-fried veggies from dinner can make a filling for an omelet in the morning. Think of leftovers as ingredients for new creations.

Properly Preserve Food

Appropriate storage techniques can significantly prolong the lifespan of your groceries. Invest in airtight containers for storing leftover meals. Keep your fridge and pantry organized so that you can easily see what you have available. Store vegetables correctly to prevent ripening or spoilage.

Embrace the Principles of "Nose to Tail" and "'Root to Stem" Cooking

These are not just ways to reduce waste, but also allow you to make the most out of every part of an animal or plant. Rather than discarding them, you can use meat bones to create a nutritious broth. Vegetable scraps such as onion skins and carrot tops can be utilized in the same manner. Additionally, leaves from vegetables like cauliflower and beets can be sautéed or added to salads for extra taste and nutrition.

Plan

Planning your meals in advance is a strategy to minimize food waste and ensure you only buy what you need. By knowing what you'll be cooking and eating for the week, you can avoid food spoiling before it gets used.

Start Composting

Consider composting if you have a garden, as it's a good way to reduce food waste and improve your soil quality. Fruit and vegetable scraps, coffee grounds, eggshells, and even yard waste can all be added to a compost pile.

It's essential to remember that every action we take to reduce food waste matters. These practices not only save money, they also have a positive impact on the environment. Let's make a commitment to waste less and nourish Glucotopia efficiently!

Comparing the Cost of Different Lifestyles

It's important to consider the expenses related to different lifestyles in order to fully understand the long-term savings associated with a healthy diet for individuals with diabetes. Let's compare a lifestyle that involves eating healthy food and exercising regularly with an unhealthy lifestyle that includes processed foods and a lack of physical activity over a period of six months.

Healthy Diet Versus Standard Diet

A healthy diet primarily consists of fruits, vegetables, lean proteins, and whole grains. While the initial cost of groceries might be higher compared to processed foods, there are benefits that come into play. For instance, reduced cravings result in less snacking and fewer expenses on eating out. While a standard diet may be cheaper in terms of grocery costs, it often leads to additional spending on snacks, fast food, and dining out.

Exercise Versus a Sedentary Lifestyle

Regular physical activity is a part of a healthy lifestyle. While there might be costs associated with gym memberships or home exercise equipment, engaging in physical activity reduces the risk of various health conditions, leading to lower health-care expenses. Conversely, leading a sedentary lifestyle may not have direct financial implications, but can contribute to various health issues that result in increased medical costs.

Medical Expenses

Living a healthy lifestyle has been linked to a decrease in the need for prescription medication. Living a healthy lifestyle, such as adopting a healthy diet and engaging in regular physical activity, can lead to a reduced reliance on medications for diabetes management. This reduction in medication usage can result in cost savings over a period of six months. Conversely, an unhealthy lifestyle often leads to an increased need for medication and frequent visits to the doctor.

Additional Expenses

Choosing a healthy lifestyle often results in improved well-being, which can reduce the need for supplementary expenses such as regular visits to chiropractors or sessions of massage therapy. Conversely, inflammation and stress resulting from an unhealthy lifestyle may necessitate frequent sessions of these treatments, thereby increasing costs.

It is important to note that these cost breakdowns are estimates and actual expenses may vary depending on circumstances, location, specific dietary requirements, and medical needs. Moreover, it is worth emphasizing that the benefits of adopting a healthy lifestyle extend beyond savings; they include enhanced quality of life, increased lifespan, and improved well-being.

Case Studies

Let's imagine this scenario: picture two neighbors, John and Sarah, both of whom are dealing with type 2 diabetes. John follows a standard diet and lifestyle while Sarah makes the decision to embrace a healthier approach.

John's Lifestyle (Standard Diet)

John allocates around $150 per week for groceries, choosing food options that are quick to prepare but often contain high sugar levels, unhealthy fats, and lectins. Additionally, his love for dining out adds $100 to his monthly expenses. Despite spending $200 per month on medication and visiting the doctor once a month for $200 per visit, he continues to experience symptoms related to his diabetes. To alleviate inflammation-induced pain, he frequently seeks physiotherapy care at a cost of $100 per session once per month. Over a six-month period, John's lifestyle ends up costing him $7,200.

Sarah's Lifestyle (Healthy Diet);

By contrast, Sarah decides to invest in groceries by spending $200 per week. She focuses on incorporating plenty of produce, proteins, and healthy oils into her diet while opting for lectin-free alternatives when possible. These new dietary habits result in reduced cravings, subsequently reducing her dine-out expenses to around $50 per month.

Switching to a healthy diet and incorporating physical activity has proven to be beneficial. As a result, her medication costs have reduced significantly to $100 per month. Not only that, she also needs fewer visits to the doctor (once every three months) and her inflammation levels have significantly decreased, leading to less frequent chiropractic visits (once every three months as well). Over the span of six months, Sarah's overall expenses related to her lifestyle amount to $5,700.

When comparing these two paths, Sarah manages to save $1,500 over six months. It's important to note that this monetary saving is only one aspect of the benefits she gains. The significant impact is on her quality of life—improved health indicators, fewer diabetes symptoms, and reduced inflammation levels, all contributing to a sense of well-being. She isn't simply surviving; she's thriving!

Although adopting a healthy lifestyle may initially seem expensive, it ultimately leads to substantial savings in the long run—both financially and in terms of health. By prioritizing her well-being and investing in her health, Sarah has not only saved money, she has also taken a significant step toward reversing her diabetes.

It's worth mentioning that individual choices, living situations, and geographic locations can greatly impact cost implications. However, this example serves as a reminder that what may appear "expensive" at first glance can actually turn out to be cost-effective when considering the bigger picture.

As our journey through Glucotopia comes to an end, one thing is evident: maintaining this vibrant and balanced city doesn't require huge amounts of money. The streets of Glucotopia are filled with foods that aren't exclusive to the wealthy few. The notion that eating healthily is expensive is simply a myth.

In reality, nourishing Glucotopia with foods packed with nutrients is achievable for everyone. It's about being a savvy shopper and understanding the value of food—its nutritional content rather than just its price tag. It's about embracing the joy of cooking at home and taking control of our health. We should make the most of what we have, minimize waste, and show respect for the resources that nourish us.

What truly matters is not how much money we spend on food, it's the value we gain from it. Our health is an investment like no other. It forms the foundation of our lives, empowering us to live, pursue our dreams, and be there for our loved ones.

So, I warmly invite you to join me in this commitment—lets prioritize our well-being by making thoughtful choices when it comes to food. Let's appreciate and respect the nourishment we provide to our bodies. Remember, each one of us holds the key to unlocking the best possible future. With these tools and strategies at hand, we are well prepared to experience a future filled with wellness, vitality, and equilibrium.

Let's not simply feed ourselves; lets truly nourish ourselves. Let's make every bite and every food choice count toward creating a Glucotopia—a place where balance, energy, and good health thrive. Because, regardless of constraints, each one of us deserves to live in their version of Glucotopia.

Chapter Fifteen

The HAPPINESS Formula

Your Key to Unlocking a More Balanced, Healthier Life

I n the heart of Glucotopia, where every street resonates with stories of triumphs and challenges, I discovered a secret—a powerful formula capable of reshaping destinies. It's not an enchantment or a forgotten potion, but rather a way of life, a rhythm, a dance of choices and habits that people embrace with every moment they are awake

I named it the HAPPINESS formula not only because the reflects the constituent parts but also because it signifies the profound transformation it brought about within me. There were days, not long ago, when the overwhelming clouds of diabetes cast shadows over all my endeavors, turning each moment into an uphill battle. Those were the days filled with uncertainty, thoughts, and questioning if happiness would ever shine upon me again.

However, as I started aligning my routines with this formula, something magical began to unfold. It felt as though I was a composer skillfully orchestrating the symphony of my life to harmonize with the beats of the HAPPINESS formula. The changes were initially subtle—like whispers at dawn, breaking through the darkness. Through dedication, unwavering determination, and steadfast commitment, these changes became more noticeable and tangible.

The components of the HAPPINESS formula are as follows:

H: Hydration—*the source of vitality*

A: Activity—*move it to lose it*

P: Pasture-raised meat, wild-caught fish, and eggs: *the "meat" of the matter*

P: Plants—more green leafy vegetables: *the heroes of our story*

I: Inflammation-free and intermittent fasting: *a key to the wellness vault*

N: Nourishing (fermented foods): *the lifeblood of Glucotopia*

E: Elimination of toxins: *the guardians of our health*

S: Sleep and Supplements: *the restorative and rejuvenating forces of Glucotopia*

S: Stress-free and Sugar-free: *the serene and sweet stance of Glucotopia*

Every morning as the sun paints its colors across Glucotopia, I wake up with a sense of excitement for the day ahead. It's not just about starting a new day, it's also about embracing a commitment to finding happiness. The HAPPINESS formula is more than a routine or some guidelines; it acts as my guiding compass in life. It's like a symphony that my heart follows, echoing in every decision and thought I make.

With each sunrise, I don't just go through the motions of my day. I embrace them wholeheartedly, adding colors from the HAPPINESS palette to every aspect of my life. From savoring water to finding solace in restful sleep, every element comes together like threads weaving a beautiful tapestry.

Gone are the times when despair and illness cast shadows on every corner. Glucotopia now shines with hope and radiates an aura of rejuvenation and vitality. As the city pulses with energy, so does my spirit—it dances with joy and revels in the freedom from ailments that once held me back.

This transformation goes beyond health improvement; it's an awakening. It's a journey of finding the truth where each moment, breath, and heartbeat resonates with the magic of the HAPPINESS formula.

There is a kind of miracle that offers more than a longer life—it promises a life lived to its fullest potential, brimming with richness and joy.

The true essence of the HAPPINESS formula lies not in comprehending its components but in integrating them into your everyday existence. It's not a passing phase or a lived resolution; it requires lifelong commitment. Imagine each element of the formula as threads and, with each day of dedication, you weave together a tapestry of well-being and resilience. I can personally attest to its potency—the more consistently you follow, it the greater the rewards. It goes beyond being a guide; it transforms your journey, standing as an indomitable defense against ailments and propelling you toward a life bursting with vitality and enthusiasm.

To those who read this, grasp the gravity of its message. This isn't just another chapter in some book—it's an invitation to embrace an extraordinary state of wellness. I stand before you not as a preacher, but as someone who has experienced firsthand the transformative power and fulfillment that comes from following the HAPPINESS formula. My own path from despair to optimum health was paved with the golden bricks of this remarkable framework.

Each day it becomes my focus, my commitment, my challenge. I reflect on the progress I've made by following it and identify areas where I can further improve. This straightforward approach has served as my road map to enhanced well-being, playing a role in reversing my diabetes.

By adhering to the principles of the HAPPINESS formula, I have experienced a transformation in both my energy levels and my overall health. It's not an abstract concept; it has become an integral part of my daily routine. As you delve into this chapter, I sincerely hope you recognize its significance well—because once you fully commit to it like I have, you'll witness genuine results. Let's embark on this journey toward health and happiness together.

This chapter symbolizes the commencement of your path toward a healthier and more content life. As we set sail on this journey, always remember that every single stride you take, regardless of its size, signifies progress. So, are you prepared to embrace the next step toward your metamorphosed life? Let's plunge into it!

Hydration: The Source of Vitality

Alright, let's delve deeper into the captivating journey of hydration! Water is more than H_2O for our bodies; it serves as a vital life force that powers our system efficiently, just like the pristine rivers flowing through our cities and keeping everything vibrant and alive.

Just like every resident of Glucotopia needs water to stay active and flourish, every single cell in our body also relies on this essential resource. Without hydration, these cells would become parched and less effective, and overall bodily functions would gradually slow down.

Hydration plays a role in a multitude of bodily functions. Did you know that 75% of our brain is made up of water? When we lack hydration, the function of our brain can decline, causing issues with thinking and reasoning. Similarly, our heart composed of 73% water, and heavily depends on proper hydration for optimal performance.

Now, let's discuss the key figure in this narrative: the mighty Kidnoid (kidneys). This vital organ filters waste from our bloodstreams, regulates electrolytes, and maintains a fluid balance. If we don't consume water, the Kidnoid has to work harder to preserve this delicate equilibrium, which over time potentially leads to harm.

This is especially important for people managing diabetes. Keeping yourself hydrated helps to lower blood sugar levels by enabling the kidneys to eliminate glucose from the body through urine. On the contrary, when we are dehydrated the liver releases glucose into the bloodstream, potentially raising blood sugar levels.

So, how can we make sure we stay properly hydrated? It's not about drinking water when you feel thirsty. By that time, your body is already a bit dehydrated. We should aim to drink a regular amount of water throughout the day to prevent dehydration.

However, it's important to remember that not all fluids are beneficial. Sugary drinks can cause an increase in blood glucose levels, while alcoholic beverages can lead to dehydration.

Instead, choose options like herbal teas, green tea, or naturally flavored water. Adding a slice of lemon or a few fresh mint leaves to your water can make it more enjoyable and encourage you to drink more throughout the day.

Let's raise our glasses (filled with water of course!) and embark on this journey of staying hydrated. It's the first step toward maintaining harmony and well-being in our "Glucotopia," our body, with the ultimate goal of achieving a happier version of yourself!

Activity: Move It to Lose It

The second component of the HAPPINESS equation is physical activity. In the world of Glucotopia, physical activity encompasses movements like jiggling, wiggling, dancing, running, and simply staying active. Just as muscle cells enjoy flexing, we too should embrace movement.

While we won't delve into the specifics as there's a dedicated chapter for that, it's important to note that physical activity doesn't necessarily entail intense gym workouts or marathon running. It can be as simple as choosing stairs over elevators, walking your dog regularly, or engaging in gardening activities. The more you move your body, the better you will feel and function.

Our bodies are naturally designed to be in motion; when they remain stagnant for long periods, they start to resist. Yes: leading a sedentary lifestyle can contribute to insulin resistance and impede the effectiveness of our helpful Insulinas. On the other hand, an active body helps keep insulin resistance at bay.

Furthermore, increasing your level of activity can aid in weight loss efforts, lower blood glucose levels, reduce stress levels, and enhance overall mood.

Pasture-Raised Meat, Wild-Caught Fish, and Eggs: The "Meat" of the Matter

When it comes to adopting a healthy diet, it's important to take a closer look at where our protein sources come from. As I started my journey, I came across terms like "pasture raised," "wild-caught," "free-range," and "cage -free." Going deeper into the subject, I discovered that these terms aren't just marketing phrases but actually represent farming practices that have significant impacts on both the nutritional value of the food and the well-being of animals.

When comparing pasture-raised meat with factory-farmed meat in terms of nutrition, there are some differences. One notable distinction is found in the fatty acid composition of the meat. Pasture-raised animals, due to their grass-based diet, produce meat that contains high levels of omega-3 fatty acids. These polyunsaturated fats are known for their heart-healthy properties. In 2010, a study comparing the nutritional profiles of grass-fed and grain-fed beef was published in the *Nutrition Journal* (Daley et al., 2010). The authors confirmed that grass-fed beef generally has a more favorable composition of fatty acids.

Specifically, they found that beef from cows fed on grass contains high levels of omega-3 fats, which are essential for our health. They offer numerous benefits, such as reducing inflammation and promoting heart health.

Furthermore, the study revealed that grass-fed beef is also richer in conjugated linoleic acid (CLA) compared to beef from grain-fed cows. CLA is a type of fat associated with health advantages, including improved body composition and potential anti-cancer properties.

These findings suggest that, although grass-fed beef may be pricier than grain-fed alternatives, the higher cost could be justified by its nutritional value. Choosing grass-fed beef could be seen as an investment in your well-being considering its long-term benefits.

Why is this significant? Omega-3 fatty acids play a key role, in our bodies as they are part of cell membranes and contribute to heart health, brain function, and reducing inflammation. Omega-3 and omega-6 fatty acids are crucial for our bodies because we cannot produce them naturally, so we need to get them from our diet. However, the standard current diet tends to have a higher amount of omega-6 fats compared to omega-3s. When omega-6 fats are consumed excessively without a balance of omega 3s, they can cause inflammation and contribute to various health issues.

Like the comparison between meat from pasture-raised animals and factory-farmed ones, it's also important to distinguish between wild-caught fish and farm-raised fish. Wild-caught fish are what their name suggests. They're caught in their natural habitats such as oceans, rivers, or lakes. In these environments they follow their usual diets, which typically consist of smaller fish and aquatic plants. This diverse diet contributes to their nutritional value.

When we consider the levels of fatty acids, wild-caught fish far outshine their farm-raised counterparts. The reason for this difference lies in their diet. Wild fish primarily consume algae and other sea plants that are rich in omega-3s, whereas farm-raised fish are often fed processed feed that's high in fat content to promote rapid growth.

In addition to the health implications, there are other factors to consider as well. Farm-raised fish are often kept in conditions that increase disease transmission and require antibiotic use. Moreover, waste from these farms can pollute surrounding waters. On the other hand, opting for wild-caught fish is a way to support sustainable fishing practices that maintain the delicate balance of marine ecosystems.

Even though wild-caught fish may come with a higher price tag, their nutritional benefits and positive environmental impact make them an important addition to a health-conscious diet. Consider including wild-caught fish in your meals a few times per month and relish not only their taste but also the health advantages they provide and their positive effect on the environment.

It's worth noting that not all fish are equal in terms of their nutritional qualities. Some species of fish contain higher levels of mercury, which is a neurotoxin, so it's advisable to consume them in moderation. Opt for low-mercury options like salmon, sardines, and trout as everyday choices, while reserving high-mercury varieties such as tuna and swordfish for occasional indulgences.

It's essential to acknowledge that the nutrient composition of eggs can differ significantly based on factors such as the chicken's diet and living conditions. In a study published in the *Renewable Agriculture and Food Systems* journal in 2010, researchers discovered significant differences in nutritional value between eggs from pasture-raised hens and those from commercially raised hens (Karsten et al., 2010).

The study showed that eggs from pasture-raised hens tend to be more nutrient rich compared to eggs from commercially raised hens. They contain as twice as much omega-3 fatty acids, which play a crucial role in brain function and reducing inflammation. Additionally, they have three times more vitamin E, an antioxidant that protects our body cells from damage, and seven times more beta carotene. Beta carotene is converted into vitamin A by our bodies, which is essential for vision, immune function, and cell growth.

What's more, eggs from pasture-raised hens were also found to contain less cholesterol and saturated fat. Although dietary cholesterol doesn't affect blood cholesterol levels as much as once thought, for individuals who are particularly sensitive, the lower cholesterol content in pasture-raised eggs may be an added advantage.

These findings underscore the fact that not all eggs are equal. The way chickens are raised and their diet can significantly influence the profile of their eggs. Therefore, if your budget permits and they are available to you, selecting eggs from pasture-raised hens can be a great choice.

However, it's crucial to keep in mind that prioritizing the optimal options within your financial means and considering what is locally accessible can still play a role in maintaining a well-rounded and nourishing diet. If pasture-raised items are not financially viable or difficult to find in your area, strive for the highest-quality products that are within your reach and budget. Achieving health and balanced nutrition is about overall eating habits rather than striving for perfection with every single decision.

Please keep in mind that when we talk about meats and poultry, we are actually comparing the benefits of pasture-raised/grass-fed meat over the conventional meat that is commonly available in stores. Therefore, it is not advisable to include even pasture-raised varieties as a dietary staple. Consuming them excessively is not beneficial for our health and a useful rule of thumb is to restrict your meat consumption to the size of your fist per portion. Our goal for meat intake is to get omega-3 and protein.

For our vegetarian friends, the key lies in making mindful and conscious choices that prioritize quality. While you will not be including pasture-raised meat or wild-caught fish in your meals, the essence here is to seek out and consume the best possible plant-based proteins. Look for hemp tofu, pressure-cooked beans, hemp seeds, and various other nuts and seeds. If eggs are part of your diet, always go for those laid by free-range or pasture-raised hens. By ensuring that the vegetarian or vegan proteins you choose are of a high quality, you're not just providing sustenance to your body; you're nurturing it in line with the principles of the HAPPINESS formula.

In essence, being a vegetarian or vegan within the HAPPINESS framework isn't about excluding certain food groups. Instead, it's about enriching your decisions to ensure that every bite resonates with a holistic approach to health and well-being. It's acknowledging that each meal presents an opportunity for nourishment, healing, and thriving. As you embark on your journey guided by the HAPPINESS formula, remember: it's not just, about what you eat but also how mindfully and ethically you choose to eat.

Plants—- More Green Leafy Vegetables: The Heroes of Our Story

Now let's move on to another character in our journey toward happiness: the second P, which represents plants, and specifically more green leafy vegetables. If we were in Glucotopia, these would be like green forests that contribute to cleaner and healthier air in the city. The powerful antioxidants and fiber found in these vegetables act as a shield against toxins and harmful substances.

Green leafy vegetables such as spinach, kale, collard greens, and Swiss chard are incredibly nutritious. They are packed with vitamins, minerals, and fiber that play a crucial role in maintaining optimal health and managing diabetes.

One of their benefits is their high dietary fiber content. This fiber helps regulate blood sugar levels by slowing down the absorption of sugar into the bloodstream. As a result, it prevents spikes in blood glucose and insulin levels. Moreover, these vegetables are rich in magnesium—a mineral often lacking in people with type 2 diabetes. Increasing magnesium intake may improve insulin resistance.

Furthermore, green leafy vegetables also play a role in maintaining a healthy gut. The dietary fiber they provide acts as fuel for our gut bacteria, promoting a beneficial microbiota.

Green leafy vegetables offer more than a direct impact on blood sugar levels and gut health. They are packed with antioxidants like vitamin C, flavonoids, and carotenoids, acting as a force against harmful free radicals and reducing oxidative stress. This is especially important because oxidative stress contributes to inflammation and various chronic diseases, including diabetes.

In addition to their antioxidant properties, green leafy vegetables are rich in potassium, which helps maintain blood pressure—a common concern for people with diabetes. They also contain high amounts of vitamin K, which plays a crucial role in blood clotting and bone health.

Furthermore, green leafy vegetables are low in calories and high in fiber, making them an excellent choice for weight management. Maintaining a healthy weight is particularly important for managing diabetes effectively while preventing related complications.

Green leafy veggies are incredibly versatile. They can be added to our meals in countless ways. Whether it's in salads, soups, green smoothies, or stir fries, there are multiple possibilities to enjoy their health benefits.

However, it's important to keep in mind that how we prepare these greens can have an impact on their nutritional value. Lightly steaming or sautéing them helps preserve their nutrients. Overcooking may cause some loss.

When it comes to leading a healthier life and managing diabetes better, these leafy greens can truly be our heroes by boosting our internal Glucotopia with their nutritional power. However, they are just one piece of the puzzle—each element of our comprehensive HAPPINESS formula plays a unique role and together they bring the most significant health benefits.

As we continue on this journey, let's not forget to appreciate the contribution of these leafy heroes before moving on to explore equally important components of our HAPPINESS formula.

Inflammation-Free and Intermittent Fasting: A Key to the Wellness Vault

There is a dedicated chapter on this topic, so we will not go into too many details here.

In the realm of our HAPPINESS formula, the letter I embodies a lifestyle that promotes freedom from inflammation. We prioritize maintaining a diet that's free from lectins and GMOs, envisioning a clean and peaceful environment in our Glucotopia cityscape, untouched by the harmful effects of pollution. Our goal is to ensure that the city's residents, our body cells, thrive in a stress-balanced environment that supports their optimal functioning.

Inflammation serves as a double-edged sword. On one side it is a necessary response of our bodies to injuries and infections—a protective mechanism aimed at healing and restoring equilibrium. However, when inflammation becomes chronic, it switches to its other edge—a harmful state that silently but steadily wreaks havoc on our overall health. It plays a role in conditions such as insulin resistance, diabetes, and various other health complications.

As we delve into embracing an inflammation free lifestyle, let us first explore lectins—proteins commonly found in grains and legumes. Although these proteins may seem innocuous at first glance, they can sometimes become culprits in damaging our gut lining and causing what is known as leaky gut. This situation leads to a series of reactions that worsen insulin resistance and contribute to various health problems.

Moving on to GMOs: while GMOs are commonly found in the food industry, their impact on our health is an ongoing subject of research. Some studies suggest a connection between consuming GMOs and increased inflammation, prompting us to consider opting for GMO foods for the sake of our well-being.

Intermittent fasting is the significant pillar of our journey. Though we've touched upon this in prior chapters, its pivotal role within the HAPPINESS formula merits further emphasis.

Intermittent Fasting is more than just a dietary plan. It's akin to the ebb and flow of tides, a rhythmic dance of feeding and fasting that aligns with our body's natural cycles. Think of it as Glucotopia's own circadian rhythm, where its inhabitants—our cells—get periods of active work, rest, and rejuvenation.

Benefits of Intermittent Fasting are multifaceted:

- **Metabolic Switch:** After certain hours of fasting, our body starts using stored fats as an energy source instead of relying on glucose. This switch promotes fat burning and aids in weight loss.

- **Insulin Sensitivity:** Regularly practicing IF can enhance the body's response to insulin, making it more efficient in transporting glucose. This is particularly invaluable for prediabetics and diabetics.

- **Cellular Repair:** During fasting, cells initiate a process called autophagy, where they remove damaged components, leading to regeneration.

- **Hormonal Balance:** IF can influence several hormones that regulate growth, stress, and metabolism, fostering a harmonious balance beneficial for overall health.

- **Mindful Eating:** By constraining eating windows, one becomes more attuned to hunger cues and satiety signals, promoting healthier food choices and mindful eating.

As we move forward, keep in mind that while Intermittent Fasting offers numerous benefits, it's essential to approach it with knowledge and understanding. Like any health regimen, its effectiveness is enhanced when tailored to individual needs, underpinned by mindfulness and consistency.

Remember, the journey through Glucotopia isn't about adhering to stringent rules but understanding and embracing practices that nourish both body and spirit. Intermittent Fasting, when approached correctly, can be one of those transformative tools.

Embarking on a journey toward an inflammation-free and intermittent fasting based lifestyle may seem challenging, especially with the prevalence of foods rich in lectins, GMOs and excessive choices in our diets. However, with each step, we take our aim is to disperse the clouds of inflammation hanging over Glucotopia and allow the sunshine of health and well-being to enter.

As we explore the components of our HAPPINESS formula together, remember that each element acts as a key that unlocks the door to wellness. Let's keep delving into these principles, gaining understanding and putting them into action as we journey toward the ultimate prize: a life filled with improved health and happiness.

Nurturing (Fermented Foods): The Essence of Glucotopia

As we delve deeper into the realm of the HAPPINESS formula, we encounter the letter N, representing nurturing, with a focus on the captivating world of fermented foods. Imagine these foods as the life force flowing through every corner and crevice of our city, infusing it with vitality, balance, and vibrancy.

Fermented foods are essentially a tribute to the wisdom passed down by our ancestors. We have covered them in detail in a previous chapter, so will just provide an overview here. Fermented foods undergo transformation by micro-organisms and are brimming with probiotics—those friendly warriors in our gut that enhance digestive health, strengthen our immune system, and contribute to a flourishing internal ecosystem. For individuals navigating the path of diabetes, fermented foods hold greater significance. Diabetes is often accompanied by imbalances in the gut, which can negatively impact blood sugar control and increase complications. By nourishing our bodies with rich fermented foods, we effectively restore equilibrium to our gut health, paving the way for improved diabetes management.

The realm of fermented foods is a tapestry woven from an array of flavors, colors, and textures. With the taste of sauerkraut, the satisfying crunch of pickles, the creamy texture of yogurt, and the slightly tart flavor of kefir, there is something to delight every palate. What's even better is that you can easily make fermented foods at home, allowing you to have complete control over the ingredients and ensuring they meet your nutritional requirements.

As we embark on this journey into the world of fermented foods, we are not only nourishing our bodies but also providing essential fuel for our cells, our gut microbiota, and our entire inner ecosystem. This balance and optimal functioning are what bring about a thriving Glucotopia—a place where happiness flourishes by embracing a rounded approach.

Elimination of Toxins: The Guardians of Our Health

Here we are, discussing the E in the formula for HAPPINESS— getting rid of harmful substances. Think of this aspect as the guardians of our community, always vigilant in safeguarding us from unwelcome intruders.

Alright, let's delve into this! Eliminating toxins—it almost sounds like a mission for a superhero, doesn't it? Well, that's what our bodies do each and every day. They work tirelessly, battling against the forces of harm and keeping us secure and in good health. Within our bodies, these superheroes take the form of detoxifying organs such as the liver, kidneys, skin, lungs, and others.

Just as even superheroes can find themselves overwhelmed when faced with an excessive number of adversaries at once, our bodies can also struggle when burdened with an overload of toxins. These harmful substances can originate from a number of sources, including the food we consume, the air we breathe, and even the products we apply to our skin.

Picture this: every time we consume processed foods that are rich in unhealthy fats, sugars, and chemicals; it's as if we're unleashing a fresh wave of villains into Glucotopia. Our hardworking detox organs have to put in a huge effort to fight against these invaders and maintain smooth functioning. Over time, this can lead to the organs becoming overburdened and less efficient.

The great news is that there are effective ways we can support our bodies in this crucial detoxification process.

Firstly, prioritize consuming whole foods whenever possible. Such foods are less likely to contain toxins and more likely to provide the necessary nutrients for optimal bodily functions.

Secondly, ensure you stay properly hydrated. Drinking a good amount of water is vital as it helps flush out toxins from our bodies. So, remember to sip water throughout the day and keep those rivers flowing smoothly!

Thirdly, incorporate physical activity into your routine. Engaging in exercise promotes circulation within the blood and lymphatic systems, aids digestion, reduces tension, and assists the body in eliminating toxins.

Another benefit to mention is that red light therapy has been found to have amazing effects on detoxifying the body. You may want to consider incorporating sauna sessions into your routine. In particular, the use of infrared saunas has shown impressive results in eliminating toxins from the body.

Lastly, pay attention to the products you use both at home and on your body. Many cleaning products and personal care items contain chemicals that contribute to our body's load.

Always remember that it's not about striving for perfection. Instead, focus on making sustainable changes that can have a significant impact in the long term.

So, are you ready to become one of the superheroes of Glucotopia? Let's embark on this journey toward a body free from toxins and a happier healthier version of yourself!

Sleep & Supplements: The Twin Restorative and Rejuvenating Forces of Glucotopia

In our ever-evolving world, where technological advancements and fast-paced lifestyles dominate, two pivotal elements of health are often overshadowed: quality sleep and nutritional balance. Our modern society, with its relentless demands and 24/7 connectivity, has unknowingly traded the serene stillness of the night and the nurturing gifts of nature for artificial lights and quick fixes. We now find ourselves caught in a paradox – the very advancements designed to enhance our lives sometimes detach us from its core essentials.

Yet, amidst this hustle and the distant hum of our bustling lives, two age-old guardians stand resilient, beckoning us back to a state of equilibrium and vitality: Sleep and Supplements. They are not mere afterthoughts or optional luxuries. They are the cornerstones of our well-being, the rhythms that align with our body's innate wisdom. By embracing and harmonizing with these twin forces, we can navigate the complexities of the modern world, fortified and rejuvenated. It's time we recognized and revered them for what they are – the silent sentinels of Glucotopia, guiding us towards a life of vibrancy, clarity, and holistic wellness.

Think of sleep as the night shift in Glucotopia, a period when the city's hustle and bustle settles down, allowing the repair crew to work their magic. During this time, our cells undergo maintenance, just like buildings being attended to, our veins and arteries (the roads) get cleared of blockages, and our metabolism (the city's energy supply) is regulated and replenished.

Our body's internal clock, known as the circadian rhythm, dictates our sleep-wake cycle. Central to this cycle are the distinct stages of sleep, particularly the Rapid Eye Movement (REM) and deep sleep stages. REM sleep is a phase where dreams are most vivid, and brain activity intensifies, closely resembling that of wakefulness. In contrast, deep sleep is when our body undergoes significant restoration; muscles are repaired, and vital processes for overall health take place. The cyclical dance between these stages not only aids in physical rejuvenation but also in mental and emotional recalibration.

When we deprive ourselves of sleep, it hampers the night shift workers in Glucotopia from completing their tasks effectively. This leads to a backlog of repairs and an inefficient energy supply system. In our bodies, it manifests as impaired insulin regulation, increased food cravings, an overactive stress response, and even unintentional weight gain.

In the context of managing diabetes, sleep plays an even more crucial role. Chronic lack of sleep can cause an increase in blood sugar levels as the body requires insulin to regulate glucose properly.

But don't worry—there's good news! We have the ability to enhance our sleep quality. By practicing sleep hygiene, we can improve both the duration and quality of our sleep. This includes maintaining a sleep schedule, creating a peaceful sleeping environment, and managing lifestyle factors like diet and exercise that affect how well we sleep.

Moreover, the benefits of sleep hygiene go beyond just regulating glucose levels. Getting enough sleep is associated with improved mood, increased energy levels, enhanced immune function, and even sharper mental clarity. It's clear that quality sleep provides benefits that extend beyond Glucotopia.

Before going to bed, it's recommended to follow a 10–3–2–1–0 rule for better sleep. First avoid consuming any caffeine at all for 10 hours before bedtime. Next, refrain from eating or drinking alcohol within 3 hours of bedtime. Additionally, try to wrap up any work-related activities at 2 hours before getting into bed. Lastly, make sure to disconnect from screens such as phones, TVs, and computers for least an hour prior to sleep (Mohamed, 2021).

In today's world, the saying "You are what you eat" takes on greater importance. However, various factors such as soil degradation, industrial farming, and GMOs have altered the nutritional profile of our foods. While our plates may be full, the essential nutrients within the food are not as dense as they once were. This discrepancy between our dietary intake and what our bodies truly need brings to light the significant role of supplements.

Diet and exercise indeed form the foundational pillars of diabetes management. However, the influence of certain minerals and vitamins, especially in maintaining glucose levels, cannot be understated.

- **Chromium:** This trace element is pivotal for improving insulin action and managing blood sugar levels. It plays a vital role in the metabolism of carbohydrates, fats, and proteins.

- **Magnesium:** Essential for multiple biochemical reactions in the body, a deficiency can impair insulin secretion. Supplementing with magnesium can assist those struggling with or at risk of diabetes.

- **Vitamin B Complex:** These vitamins are often reduced when taking certain medications for lowering glucose levels.

Ensuring adequate intake of B vitamins is important for maintaining energy levels and metabolic health. Also most of the B complexes are produced by our healthy gut bacteria. If there is a deficiency of Vitamin B, chances are that there is a depletion in healthy bacteria load in your gut.

- **Alpha-lipoic acid:** This powerful antioxidant is known for its potential to minimize the symptoms of nerve damage in diabetes and aid in glucose utilization.

- **Berberine:** Derived from various plants, berberine has shown potential in reducing blood sugar levels and improving overall metabolic health.

- **Curcumin:** Found in turmeric, this compound has anti-inflammatory properties and can play a role in lowering blood sugar levels.

- **Glucosamine:** Often associated with joint health, glucosamine can act as a lectin defense, protecting the body from these harmful proteins.

- **Cinnamon:** Beyond its fragrant appeal, cinnamon can have a positive effect on blood sugar regulation.

- **Probiotics:** These beneficial bacteria play a crucial role in gut health, which has been linked to improved metabolic functions and better glucose control.

The vast realm of supplements can be overwhelming, making it essential to discern quality and efficacy. When looking for effective supplements, it's crucial to opt for plant-based ones, ensuring they align with a holistic approach to health.

Purity is key. Top-tier supplements are devoid of detrimental fillers and contaminants. The source of these supplements also matters; plant-derived and ethically sourced ingredients ensure both sustainability and potency. Transparency is a hallmark of trustworthy supplement brands. From sourcing to third-party testing results, brands should willingly share detailed information.

Furthermore, the addition of supplements like berberine, curcumin, glucosamine (for lectin defense), cinnamon, and probiotics underscores the comprehensive nature of this health approach. Especially noteworthy is the emphasis on plant-based supplements, which ensures that the body is receiving nutrition in its most natural form.

In conclusion, supplements, when chosen with care and discernment, can be powerful allies in our health journey. Complementing our diets with these nutrients ensures a comprehensive approach to well-being, enhancing our body's capacity to function optimally.

Stress-free and Sugar-free: The Serene and Sweet Stance of Glucotopia

Finally, we reach the last element of the HAPPINESS equation—a stress-free existence. In Glucotopia, prioritizing peace and tranquility is of the utmost importance. Excessive conflict and tension can disrupt the functioning of the city, giving rise to a host of issues.

Similarly, within our bodies chronic stress can wreak havoc. Hormones like cortisol, which are released during periods of stress, can cause an increase in blood sugar levels and eventually lead to insulin resistance. In Glucotopia, it feels as if its inhabitants are in a state of panic, while the city's infrastructure struggles to cope with the strain.

We have a dedicated chapter for that too.

In today's dietary landscape, sugar is everywhere. When we greet the day with a bowl of cereal or sip on our mid-morning latte, we're often unwittingly consuming more sugar than we realize. Beyond the obvious culprits like candies and pastries, sugar has infiltrated our dressings, bread, sauces, and those 'health' bars we grab for convenience. The modern food industry, in its quest for longer shelf lives and enhanced taste, leans heavily on sugar. Such a pervasive presence makes it challenging to discern and control our daily sugar intake, inadvertently placing our health at risk.

While sugar tempts our taste buds with instant gratification, it silently cause wide destruction on our internal health. The fleeting energy surge it provides quickly plummets, leaving us fatigued and seeking another sugar fix. But there's more than just the energy rollercoaster. Chronic sugar consumption disrupts insulin function, laying the foundation for type 2 diabetes. It also ignites inflammation, a silent destroyer linked to a plethora of health issues from heart diseases to cancer. Over time, the sweet indulgence transforms into a potential medical crisis.

AHA suggests that we should not consume more 60 teaspoons of sugar everyday and this includes sugar from all of our resources including milk products, vegetables, and fruit as well as free sugars and I am talking about the indivduals who are non diabetics. But in this day and age, our average consumption of sugar everyday is about staggering 26 teaspoons per day. How problematic it is for the individuals with type 2 diabetes and pre-diabetes to consume that much of sugar every day?

Transitioning to a sugar-free lifestyle doesn't necessarily mean bidding farewell to sweetness. Nature provides a bounty of alternatives that can satisfy our sweet tooth without the detrimental health effects associated with refined sugars. Stevia, derived from the leaves of the Stevia plant, offers sweetness without calories. Monk fruit sweetener, made from monk fruit extract, is another zero-calorie sweetener that's grown in popularity. And then there's raw honey, a natural sweetener filled with enzymes, antioxidants, and nutrients. While it does contain sugars, its natural composition and health benefits make it a preferable option in moderation. When selecting these alternatives, it's crucial to ensure they're pure and free from added sugars or artificial components.

There are other alternatives too like erythritol, xylitol and my favorite allulose.

Allulose, also known as D-psicose, is a rare sugar found naturally in small quantities in certain fruits like figs, jackfruit, and raisins. Structurally, it's very similar to fructose, one of the main sugars found in fruits. However, what sets allulose apart is its unique metabolic pathway.

Unlike regular sugars, allulose contributes almost zero calories. It is absorbed by the body but not metabolized, meaning it's excreted largely unchanged in the urine. This unique trait makes it an appealing choice for those monitoring their calorie intake. Allulose has minimal impact on blood glucose levels, making it a safer alternative for those trying to manage their blood sugar. Preliminary allulose may play a role in improving insulin sensitivity, a vital aspect for diabetics. Improved insulin sensitivity means that the body requires less insulin to move glucose from the bloodstream into cells.

While these alternatives present many benefits, it's essential to be aware of certain aspects. In some individuals, excessive consumption can cause digestive discomfort. Just because these are some better alternatives doesn't mean they should be consumed without restraint. Moderation is key.

The Unwavering Power of the HAPPINESS Formula: A Blueprint for Transformative Success

In the vast canvas of life, with its myriad choices, anything that does not align with this formula doesn't find a place in my itinerary. It serves as my steadfast compass amidst the ever-changing winds of life's challenges. This formula, dear friends, is my unwavering guideline, my beacon, ensuring I remain firmly anchored to my true purpose.

Now, I want to speak candidly to you. There might be a day where you're tempted to stray from this path. A cheat day, perhaps. While a single detour might seem inconsequential, be wary of the message it sends to your psyche. Sure, once might not derail your progress, but it plants a seed of compromise. Over time, that seed can grow, leading to a forest of old habits, pushing you back into patterns you desperately sought to change. It's not just about the one-time action; it's about the negative feedback loop it kickstarts in your brain.

Consider this formula as more than a dietary or lifestyle choice. It's a pact, a commitment you make with yourself. An unwavering promise to honor, respect, and nurture your well-being. The HAPPINESS formula offers clarity amidst chaos, but it requires dedication. So, when you're tempted to deviate, remember why you started.

Three months. That's my challenge to you. Three months of pure dedication to this formula. The changes awaiting you aren't just physical. They're transformative, affecting your mind, spirit, and overall life's vigor.

In our existence's grand narrative, amidst life's cacophony, the HAPPINESS formula stands as a beacon. With it, you possess the ultimate roadmap, leading you towards unparalleled vitality and profound happiness.

So, as you embark on this path, remember: occasional detours might seem harmless, but they erode the commitment. Stay the course, stay steadfast, and the rewards will be manifold. It's not just about a healthier body; it's about a life inspired with purpose, joy, and an undying zest for excellence. Commit to the HAPPINESS formula, let it reshape you, and witness the dawn of your most radiant self. Because, my friends, the life of your dreams is not miles away; it's just a formula away.

For example, when I go grocery shopping, I follow the Happiness formula. First, I begin in the produce section, where I select a variety of vegetables with a particular focus on dark leafy greens. After that, I move on to the meat section, where I look for labels indicating that the meat is raised in pastures. Then I make my way to the fermented foods section, choosing items such as sauerkraut, aged cheeses, or kimchi that offer beneficial probiotics.

I am careful to read labels and ensure that the products I choose have no harmful preservatives and no GMOs. Additionally, I avoid products with added sugars, opting instead for natural sources of sweetness like organic fruits. By doing this, I ensure that the foods I consume nourish my body while keeping inflammation and toxins at bay.

When it comes to staying hydrated, carrying a water bottle has become second nature to me. Throughout the day, it has become habitual for me to refill my bottle several times. As for staying active, incorporating movement into my routine has been key—whether it's taking stairs instead of elevators or going for walks during my lunch breaks.

To promote quality sleep at night, creating a soothing sleep environment at home has been essential for me. Additionally, sticking to a bedtime routine ensures that each night is filled with restful sleep.

To cope with stress, I've integrated mindfulness practices into my routine, which helps me remain centered and composed even when faced with challenges.

The HAPPINESS Formula has had a huge impact on my life. Not only has it aided in managing my diabetes, but it has also significantly enhanced my overall well-being. However, it's crucial to acknowledge that this formula doesn't take a one-size-fits-all approach. We all possess bodies with distinct requirements. What worked for me might not work universally. Nevertheless, I firmly believe that the fundamental principles of this formula—hydration, balanced nutrition, regular exercise, sufficient sleep, and effective stress management—are universal components of a healthy lifestyle.

Understanding the HAPPINESS formula is the beginning. The next step involves incorporating it into your life in a way that aligns with your needs and lifestyle. It's about piecing together all the elements to create an image of optimal well-being.

In the next chapter, ""we will explore practical ways to integrate the HAPPINESS formula into your daily routine. We'll delve into how you can weave these principles into your everyday life, fostering balance, health, and happiness.

The path toward health is well within your grasp. The decision lies in your hands. Are you prepared to take that leap? Here's to a life filled with vitality and joy. Welcome aboard as we embark on the final stage of our journey through Glucotopia!

Chapter Sixteen

The HAPPINESS Schedule

A Guide to Balanced Living

W elcome to the next chapter of our journey through Gluco-topia, a transformative path toward a healthier and happier life. In the previous chapter we explored the different components of the HAPPINESS formula, understanding their roles, importance, and how they work together to promote optimal health. Now it's time to bring all these elements together into a plan—your personal HAPPINESS schedule.

If learning about health principles is like discovering a treasure map, then putting those principles into action is the exciting adventure that leads to finding the treasure itself. In our case, that treasure is Glucotopia—a state of health, vitality, and happiness.

Knowing these principles is only part of the challenge. The real test lies in implementing them into our lives. That's exactly what we will focus on in this chapter.

Making lasting changes in life can sometimes seem overwhelming—especially when it comes to lifestyle adjustments. You may find yourself filled with excitement at the beginning, only to feel overwhelmed by the scale of the changes you're trying to make. The path to embracing the HAPPINESS formula is no exception. However, it's important to remember that this is not about completely upending your life overnight; it's about gradually transforming, where each small change has a powerful impact that extends toward a healthier and happier future.

When I embarked on my journey to adopt the HAPPINESS formula I encountered various obstacles—figuring out how to incorporate each element into my daily routine, dealing with setbacks, and staying motivated amid the demands of everyday life. With every obstacle I overcame, I grew stronger, more resilient, and more dedicated to my well-being. I want to reassure you that you too can overcome any challenges that arise along your path, and I am here to support you through each step of this journey.

In this chapter, we will explore how to create your HAPPINESS schedule while ensuring a balance among all the essential components of the HAPPINESS formula. We will also delve into strategies for overcoming challenges and maintaining motivation.

Remember, the objective isn't to create a timetable but rather to cultivate a well-rounded and satisfying lifestyle that takes care of your body, stimulates your mind, and brings peace to your soul. As we move forward, always remember that progress is the goal, not perfection. Now, let's embark on this journey of implementing the HAPPINESS formula!

Maintaining Balance Among the Elements of the HAPPINESS Formula

Like an orchestra creating a harmonious symphony, each element of the HAPPINESS formula needs to work together in perfect balance. It's not one instrument playing too loudly while others are silenced; it's about every instrument playing its role and contributing to the overall melody. Similarly, implementing the HAPPINESS formula involves finding a balance rather than excessively focusing on one element at the expense of others.

Let's consider "Activity" and "Sleep" as an example. While regular physical activity is vital for health, pushing yourself too hard without giving your body sufficient rest can lead to burnout and hinder progress. On the other hand, quality sleep is equally essential as it allows your body to repair and rejuvenate itself. However, excessive sleep or spending hours in bed without actually sleeping can result in lethargy and various health issues.

Finding the equilibrium between maintaining proper hydration and getting rid of toxins is another important aspect to consider. It's essential to drink water to help flush out toxins from your body. However, if the water you consume is contaminated with toxins, you could unknowingly be increasing your toxin load rather than eliminating it.

These examples highlight the significance of balance. The HAPPI-NESS formula isn't about extremes, but rather about finding harmony among its various components.

It's crucial to remember that each person is unique, and so is their journey toward health and happiness. Pay attention to your body and its signals. If something doesn't feel right, don't hesitate to make adjustments in your routine or seek guidance. The HAPPINESS formula serves as a guide rather than an inflexible rulebook.

Ultimately, it's about building a way of life that not only improves your physical well-being but also nurtures your inner self and brings you happiness. As we embark on the next sections, you'll discover more insights and practical suggestions to help you strike this equilibrium and create your own unique symphony of HAPPINESS!

Overcoming Challenges and Staying Motivated

Just like any major lifestyle change, adopting the HAPPINESS approach will come with its fair share of challenges. You may encounter obstacles, face setbacks, or sometimes even feel like you're not progressing enough. This is completely normal. Remember that change is a process, not an event. The key lies in anticipating these challenges, devising strategies to overcome them, and staying committed to your journey toward well-being and contentment.

Setting Goals

A common pitfall is setting unrealistic goals that can lead to disappointment and loss of motivation when they aren't achieved. The HAPPINESS formula isn't about striving for perfection; it's about making progress. Start with goals that are achievable. For example, if you're new to activity, aiming for 30 minutes of exercise every day might seem overwhelming. Instead, begin with a 10-minute walk each day. Gradually increase the duration as your fitness improves.

Monitoring Progress

Keeping track of your progress can be a source of motivation. Consider keeping a journal to track your activities, meals, sleep patterns, and how you feel both physically and emotionally. It's a way to reflect on your progress and the positive changes you've made in your life.

Remember the importance of social support. Don't underestimate the power of having friends, family, or a supportive community by your side. Sharing your goals with them, celebrating achievements together, and relying on their encouragement during tough times can greatly boost your motivation.

Handling setbacks is part of the journey. With careful planning and good intentions, there might be occasions where you deviate from your plan to find happiness. It's okay if you miss a few workout sessions, indulge in some unhealthy meals, or experience inadequate sleep. Don't dwell on these slipups, as they don't define your progress. Instead, view them as learning experiences. Identify what led to the setback and find ways to prevent it in the future. Then pick up where you left off and continue moving.

Don't forget to celebrate every victory, no matter how small or unnecessary you might feel it is. Did you consistently get sleep for an entire week? Have you successfully incorporated leafy greens into your meals? Take the time to acknowledge these accomplishments and give yourself a well-deserved reward. They serve as evidence of your dedication to your well-being and contentment. Don't forget, it's these victories that accumulate and lead to significant transformations over time.

Sustaining a Positive Mindset

Ultimately, maintaining a positive mindset is crucial for staying motivated. Remind yourself of the reasons why you initially embarked on this journey. Envision your aspirations and the advantages you'll gain from embracing a happier lifestyle.

This journey you're on is a testament to your self-love and your commitment to your well-being. So, keep going, stay positive, and know that every step you take brings you closer to the health and happiness you deserve.

Now that we've discussed the significance of implementing the HAPPINESS formula, balancing its elements, and overcoming obstacles, let's delve into something more tangible: a 28-day guide designed to help you initiate the process.

Remember, this guide is merely a starting point. It's crucial to adapt it according to your individual needs, preferences, and daily routine. The objective isn't rigidly adhering to it, but rather using it as a foundation for incorporating the HAPPINESS principles into your everyday life.

In this guide, you'll find a plan that covers all the aspects of the HAPPINESS formula. It provides a range of recommendations for each component, including tips on diet, physical activity, stress management, and improving sleep habits.

Every day presents a chance to make decisions. You can try exploring fermented foods, adding a meditation session to your morning routine, or replacing your usual store-bought snack with a homemade option that's packed with nutrients.

Unleashing Your Potential: A 28-Day Expedition to Wellness and Joy

Embarking on a voyage toward lasting well-being and contentment requires more than simply finding the path; it calls for taking action, staying committed, and being patient. Without putting into practice what we've learned, transformation remains an aspiration.

I therefore offer you a carefully crafted 28-day blueprint that captures the essence of the HAPPINESS formula. This plan isn't a routine but rather a flexible framework that can be tailored to suit your individual lifestyle and preferences. Its purpose is to guide you in instilling habits, allowing you to witness firsthand the profound impact these changes can have on your well-being and sense of fulfillment.

This expedition may undoubtedly present challenges along the way, but it is equally poised to bring rewards. As you progress through these four weeks, subtle shifts will become evident in your health, energy levels, mood, and overall perspective on life. You will start uncovering the potential within yourself to manifest wellness and happiness.

Every day throughout this 28-day program has a focus and theme, ensuring that your journey remains dynamic and exhilarating. While the initial two weeks establish a foundation by introducing daily practices aligned with the HAPPINESS formula, the subsequent two weeks delve even deeper. They incorporate elements of diversity, challenges, and exploration to make your journey engaging and pleasurable.

Remember, the goal here isn't to reach the end of these 28 days; it's about embracing a lifestyle that nurtures you long after this four-week period. This 28-day plan is merely the beginning—a stepping stone toward a lifetime of well-being and contentment.

So, are you prepared to take that leap? Are you ready to unlock your potential and transform your life? The following pages hold the answers. Let's turn over a new leaf together, step into this thrilling new chapter, and embark on this 28-day voyage towards wellness and happiness.

Day 1 – Day 14: General Daily Plan

- **Good Morning Sunshine (6 a.m. – 7 a.m.):** Wake up feeling fresh and ready for a great day. Measure your weight and waist to keep track. Then, mix a tablespoon of inulin, a teaspoon of MCT oil with lemon water to wake up your tummy and get ready for the day. Stretch a little or do some easy yoga to get moving. Sit quietly for a bit to get your mind ready for what's coming up.

- **Keep it Light (7 a.m. – 11 a.m.):** Stick to water or herbal tea in the morning. It keeps you clear-headed for work or fun stuff you're doing. Every hour, take just five minutes to chill and reset.

- **Lunchtime (11 a.m.):** Shake up a yummy green smoothie with lots of leafy stuff, avocado, and a squeeze of lemon. It's like a salad you can drink! It might not taste great but you will be able to acquire taste in just couple of days, trust me!

- **Noontime Eats (1 p.m. – 2 p.m.):** Lunch is whatever you're in the mood for – a chicken salad or a bowl of veggie stew. After eating, go for a little walk or just take it easy for a while.

- **Afternoon Snack (4 p.m.):** When you're a bit hungry, grab some nuts or cucumber slices with guacamole. Just make sure top consume cucumbers without peels and seeds, they are full of lectins. Stretch your legs and relax for a bit.

- **Get Moving (5 p.m. – 6 p.m.):** Now's the time to get your body moving. You can pick anything that feels fun – dancing, walking, or a game of soccer with friends.

- **Dinner Time (6 p.m. – 7 p.m.):** Dinner is a nice time to slow down. Make a tasty meal with veggies and some good protein. Then just chill and enjoy your evening.

- **Evening Wind-Down:** After dinner, do what you love. Read, listen to music, or sip a cup of tea outside. It's all about feeling calm and happy before bed.

- **Weekly Win:** At the end of the week, give yourself a pat on the back for all the good things you've done for yourself. Every day in Glucotopia is a step toward feeling awesome!

Day 15 – Day 28: Enhanced Daily Plan

- **Rise and Shine (6 a.m. – 7 a.m.):** Keep up with your morning drink and quiet time. Spice it up with different stretches or yoga moves to keep it fun and work new muscles.

- **Focused Mornings (7 a.m. – 11 a.m.):** Continue your fast, drink plenty of fluids, and set your sights on doing one big task really well during these hours.

- **Smoothie Twist (11 a.m.):** Add a new surprise to your smoothies, like a pinch of cinnamon or some spirulina, to mix it up and keep your taste buds guessing.

- **Lunch Adventures (1 p.m. – 2 p.m.):** Shake up your lunch routine with new tasty recipes that are still good for you. Try flavors from around the world to make lunchtime an adventure.

- **Snack and Stretch (4 p.m – 5pm.):** Enjoy your regular snack time and maybe try an almond milk pudding for a change. Pick a new way to get active this afternoon – something fun you haven't done before.

- **Dinner Discoveries (6 p.m. – 7 p.m.):** Bring new proteins to your plate this week. Ever tried omega-3-rich fish or a new vegan protein? Now's the time!

- **Peaceful Evenings:** After dinner, make memories with family or friends, get lost in a good book, or unwind with a hobby. Also, start a bedtime routine that helps you sleep better, like saying no to phones in the bedroom.

Mapping Your Four-Week Transformation

Embarking on a journey of transformation requires a road map. Just like a traveler plans their route, considering the destinations, pit stops and landscapes, we too must strategize our path toward health and happiness. What you're about to read is a 28-day guide designed to incorporate the principles of the HAPPINESS formula into your daily life.

Each day introduces an activity or small adjustment to your routine. These actions are not random but carefully chosen to align with the core elements of the HAPPINESS formula. They serve as building blocks, helping you establish a foundation for a sustainable and healthier lifestyle.

Here's how to make use of this plan:

Consistency: Strive to follow each day's activity as closely as possible. Remember, it's not about achieving perfection but maintaining consistency.

Adaptation: Feel free to swap days or modify activities according to your comfort and convenience while avoiding skipping them altogether.

Awareness: As you progress through each day, be mindful of how these changes affect your mood, energy levels, and overall well-being. It's all part of the learning process.

Journaling: Keep a journal where you can record your experiences, challenges confronted, and victories achieved.

Not only will this serve as a way for you to reflect, but it will also provide you with the motivation you need. Now, let's delve into the four-week road map that will help you start, improve, intensify, and, ultimately, optimize your path toward becoming an healthier version of yourself.

Week 1: Initiation and Observation

- **Day 1:** Today, I will note my weight, waist circumference, mood, blood sugar level, and blood pressure as a starting point. I will drink at least 8–10 glasses of water.

- **Day 2:** Today, I will incorporate a 30-minute brisk walk into my routine.

- **Day 3:** Today, I will introduce a 12/12 intermittent fasting regime, eating within a 12-hour window.

- **Day 4:** Today, I will add one more serving of green leafy vegetables to at least one of my meals.

- **Day 5:** Today, I will ensure that 80% of my meals are made from unprocessed foods.

- **Day 6:** Today, I will include fermented foods like yogurt in my diet.

- **Day 7:** Today, I will check my weight, waist circumference, mood, blood sugar level, and blood pressure to track my progress.

Week 2: Enhancing the Regimen

- **Day 8:** Today, I will shift to an 8/16 intermittent fasting regime.

- **Day 9:** Today, I will try a new stress-relieving activity.

- **Day 10:** Today, I will create a consistent sleep schedule, aiming for 7–9 hours of sleep.

- **Day 11:** Today, I will cook a recipe using pasture-raised meats or eggs, or try a new vegetarian/vegan recipe.

- **Day 12:** Today, I will completely eliminate added sugars in any form from my diet.

- **Day 13:** Today, I will increase my physical activity to 45 minutes.

- **Day 14:** Today, I will reassess my weight, waist circumference, mood, blood sugar level, and blood pressure.

Week 3: Intensifying the Effort
- **Day 15:** Today, I will include two servings of leafy green vegetables in my meals.

- **Day 16:** Today, I will increase my physical activity to 60 minutes.

- **Day 17:** Today, I will try a new recipe that is rich in healthy fats like avocados or nuts.

- **Day 18:** Today, I will practice mindful eating, focusing on the nutritional value of my food.

- **Day 19:** Today, I will spend time in nature to enhance my mood and stress levels.

- **Day 20:** Today, I will include a serving of omega-3-rich foods like fish in my diet.

- **Day 21:** Today, I will review my progress again, using the same metrics as Day 1.

Week 4: Optimizing and Future Planning
- **Day 22:** Today, I will start the day with a glass of warm lemon water to boost digestion.

- **Day 23:** Today, I will introduce strength training exercises into my routine.

- **Day 24:** Today, I will plan meals for the next week, ensuring they align with my nutritional needs.

- **Day 25:** Today, I will practice deep breathing exercises for stress relief.

- **Day 26:** Today, I will explore new sources of plant-based proteins.

- **Day 27:** Today, I will prepare a new fermented food dish at home.

- **Day 28:** Today, I will reassess my progress and set goals for the next month.

Remember, this is just a suggested plan and can be modified according to your personal preferences and health conditions. The ultimate goal is to make lifestyle changes that are sustainable in the long term and contribute positively to your health and happiness. So, are you ready to embark on this exciting four-week transformation? Your path to health and happiness starts here!

As we draw to the close of this chapter, I want to reassure you that this journey you are about to embark on is not one of stringent rules and rigid timetables. It's a journey of exploration and learning. It's about understanding the principles of the HAPPINESS formula and how to integrate them into your lifestyle in a way that feels natural and sustainable.

Remember, the goal of this 28-day plan is not to attain perfection. We are all human, and there will be days when we might stray from our planned schedule. The key here is not to get disheartened or to give up. Instead, view such instances as opportunities to learn more about yourself, about what works for you and what doesn't, and to use this knowledge to refine your HAPPINESS schedule.

This journey is about consistent progress, not about immediate results. It's about taking small, steady steps each day toward a healthier, happier you. It's about embracing the philosophy of living in harmony with our bodies, our minds, and our environments.

Tips and Tricks for Maintaining the HAPPINESS Lifestyle

The beauty of the HAPPINESS formula lies in its flexibility. No matter what your circumstances are, you can seamlessly incorporate these principles into your life. Let's explore how individuals from all walks of life can integrate the formula into their lifestyles:

Busy Professionals

If you have a demanding career, efficiency becomes paramount. Consider dedicating time on weekends to meal prepping so that you have meals available throughout the week. Take advantage of breaks during the day to practice mindfulness or engage in bursts of physical activity, like walking or climbing stairs. Incorporate physical movement into your commute by walking or cycling whenever possible or even getting off transportation one stop early to add extra steps.

Stay-at-Home Parents

As a stay-at-home parent, your schedule may revolve around your children's needs. Try to engage in physical activity with your kids, whether that's a dance-off in the living room or a game of tag in the backyard. Encourage them to participate in meal preparation as a way to learn and ensure that wholesome homemade meals are enjoyed together. Utilize nap times or when your children are at school for mindfulness practices or to squeeze in a workout session.

Students

Being a student often means juggling classes and study sessions throughout the day. Make the most out of your schedule by incorporating activities that you find enjoyable. You can join a college sports team or make use of the campus gym. Opt for healthy options at the cafeteria, or learn to cook simple, nutritious meals at home. Don't forget to include breaks during your study schedule for workouts or mindfulness practices.

Seniors

For seniors it becomes more important to prioritize health. Consider adding exercises like walking and relaxation into your routine. Engaging in community activities can provide interaction and mental stimulation. Focus on maintaining a diet that meets all your needs and don't forget about the importance of sleep and rest. Additionally, finding relaxation in activities such as reading, painting or gardening can be beneficial.

Remember that these are just examples and the HAPPINESS formula is adaptable based on your needs and lifestyle. The goal is to integrate habits into your day in a way that feels natural and enjoyable to you. Be creative, try different strategies, and make the HAPPINESS formula personalized for yourself, because ultimately the journey toward health and happiness is yours.

Embracing Challenges and Celebrating Progress

Just like any journey, the path to living a HAPPINESS lifestyle will come with its fair share of bumps and turns. You may encounter challenges that put your determination to the test, days when motivation wanes, and moments when old habits tempt you. That's perfectly normal. Every worthwhile journey has its challenges. What truly matters is how we face those challenges head on and continue moving.

Here are some common hurdles you might encounter, along with strategies to overcome them:

Difficulty in Changing Eating Habits

Modifying habits can be quite a task, especially when it involves giving up foods you adore. However, remember that every small change makes a difference. Begin by taking small steps, such as incorporating one nutritious food into your diet each week, or eliminating one unhealthy item. Over time, as your taste buds adjust and you experience the benefits, making healthier choices will become easier.

Finding Time for Exercise

In our busy lives, finding time for exercise may sometimes feel like a challenge. Try integrating movement into your routine. Take the stairs instead of the elevator, squeeze in a quick workout during TV commercial breaks, or have a fun dance session while preparing dinner. Remember, every bit of movement contributes toward your goals.

Having Trouble Falling Asleep

Many of us struggle with quieting our minds at the end of the day. If you find yourself in this situation, try establishing a soothing bedtime routine. You could consider activities like reading a book, listening to calming music, or practicing a guided relaxation exercise. Additionally, creating an environment that promotes sleep is essential. Think about keeping the room dark, quiet, and cool.

Managing Stress

Managing stress is key to your journey toward happiness. It's important to note that stress itself isn't always negative; it's how we handle it that makes all the difference. Explore stress relief techniques to discover what works best for you. It can be anything from breathing and yoga to engaging in activities like painting or enjoying your favorite music.

While it's crucial to navigate these challenges, don't forget to celebrate your progress along the way. Every step you take toward a healthier lifestyle, no matter how small it may seem, is worth acknowledging as a victory. Opted for a salad rather than a burger? That's definitely something to cheer about! Took a five-minute relaxation break during a hectic day? That's a win! By celebrating these small wins, you're not just boosting your motivation but also enjoying the journey toward health and happiness.

Remember, living a happy lifestyle doesn't mean striving for perfection; it's, about embracing imperfections and finding contentment along the way. It's all about striving for progress, aiming to improve your health and happiness a little bit each day. So, embrace the challenges that come your way, celebrate the victories you achieve, and cherish every moment of this journey toward a happier version of yourself.

Now, as you stand on the cusp of this life-changing journey, I encourage you to take the leap. Embrace the principles outlined in the HAPPINESS formula. Integrate them seamlessly into your life. You'll witness how they gradually uplift your well-being and overall happiness.

As you move forward along this path, remember that this book will always be here to guide you. It will provide information, inspire you, and offer support as you pursue health and happiness. Look back to the chapters that delve deeper into each element of the HAPPINESS formula. They will provide detailed guidance, practical strategies, and helpful resources.

The next phase of our adventure takes us into the heart of the HAPPINESS formula, where every principle comes alive. This is where knowledge transforms into action and small changes blossom into a version of yourself. Are you ready to embark on this transformative journey?

In the wonderful words of Lao Tzu, "The journey of a thousand miles begins with a step." Begin your journey toward a happier life today. Remember, the only thing holding you back from achieving health and happiness is taking that first step. Let's progress together one day at a time as we navigate through the city of Glucotopia and embrace a life filled with vitality and joy. Onwards and upwards!

Chapter Seventeen

Harnessing Technology for Health

Your Essential Happiness App

I n today's world, technology plays a central role in our daily lives. It has revolutionized how we work, communicate, and take care of our well-being. Understanding the potential of digital tools to support your journey toward managing diabetes, we've made the decision to bring the HAPPINESS formula right to your fingertips.

This section introduces our forthcoming application, a companion crafted to help you maintain focus, organization, and motivation throughout your path to improved health. The application will consolidate all the ideas, strategies, and schedules discussed in the book, making them easily accessible and simple to put into practice.

The HAPPINESS App: Key Features and Benefits

- **Personalized Profiles:** Upon registration, you'll have the opportunity to create a customized profile. The app will consider factors such as your age, weight, lifestyle choices, and diabetes status to provide tailored recommendations and monitor your progress.

- **Daily Schedules & Reminders:** No need for you to keep everything in mind. The app will house your routine while offering reminders for important tasks, like staying hydrated, having meals on time, engaging in exercise, or relaxation techniques—activities that align with the HAPPI-NESS principles.

- **Progress Tracking:** The app will allow you to log health indicators like weight measurements, waist circumference, mood changes, blood sugar levels, blood pressure readings, among others so that you can monitor your progress effectively. Using charts and graphs you can easily visualize your progress over time.

- **Goal Setting:** Following the SMART approach, the app will allow you to set daily, weekly, or monthly goals. When you achieve these goals, the app will provide reinforcement to boost your motivation.

- **Resources & Support:** The app will offer a range of resources, such as articles, videos, recipes, and exercise guides. It will also include a community feature where users can share their experiences and support one another.

- **Integration with Devices:** The app will seamlessly sync with devices to automatically track and update your physical activity and sleep data.

- **Healthcare Provider Access:** With your permission, the app can share your progress with your health-care provider. This enables them to provide care tailored to your needs.

Getting Access to the HAPPINESS App

We are currently working on bringing this application to life. If you're interested in accessing it once its ready, simply leave your email address and we will notify you once it is ready. The link is www.glutop.com.

Rest assured that you will be among the first to enjoy this tool designed to make your health journey more manageable and enjoyable.

Embracing the Digital Age for Health

In this era, it's time we embrace the potential of technology not only for convenience but also for our well-being. Through the utilization of the HAPPINESS app, our aim is to bridge the gap between knowledge and action, making it simpler than ever for individuals to adopt a lifestyle that can potentially reverse type 2 diabetes.

By incorporating the principles of the HAPPINESS formula into a user-friendly, easily accessible format, we can stay connected, committed, and on track toward achieving our health goals. Let's not forget that consistency is key throughout this journey—while the app serves as a tool, it's ultimately up to each individual to drive change.

As we navigate through this era of innovation, the realm of health and wellness continues to undergo advances. The emergence of health and wellness applications has revolutionized how we approach our well-being by empowering us with tools to effectively manage and enhance our health.

Chapter Eighteen

Your Journey, Your Pace, Your Glucotopia

As we approach the end of this book, it's time to pause and reflect on the journey we've taken together. Every chapter, every page, and every word were carefully crafted with one goal in mind: to empower you to take charge of your health and happiness, to provide you with the tools to manage your diabetes, and, ultimately, to guide you toward the path of sustainable wellness.

Your engagement with this book signifies an important first step, a commitment to self-improvement, and an investment in your health. For that, I am grateful and admire your courage. After all, it's not easy to initiate change, especially when it comes to deeply ingrained lifestyle habits.

Through the course of this book, we explored the HAPPINESS formula—a multidimensional approach to holistic well-being that underscores the profound connection between lifestyle factors and health outcomes. From hydration and air to nutrition, physical activity, sleep, stress management, and emotional wellbeing, each element of this formula embodies a piece of the puzzle in diabetes management and overall wellness.

It's important to remember, though, that the wisdom encapsulated in these pages is more than just theoretical knowledge. It's a practical guide, a road map that is intended to be used, followed, and incorporated into the daily rhythms of your life. By actively engaging with the HAPPINESS formula, you're not only expanding your understanding but also progressively nurturing a healthier, more fulfilling lifestyle.

As we move forward, let's revisit the key concepts, consolidate our understanding, and mentally prepare to turn these principles into action. Because the real journey begins not just with understanding the path, but with the courage to walk it, one step at a time.

As we continue to explore the realms of the HAPPINESS formula, it's essential to remember that this journey is deeply personal and unique to each one of us. Just as we all have different likes, dislikes, strengths, and challenges, our paths toward health and happiness will vary. And that's not just okay; it's beautiful. It adds a touch of individuality to the universal quest for health and happiness.

When embarking on this journey, it's vital to pace yourself according to your comfort and capacity. There's no need to rush or to compare your progress with others. This isn't a race; it's a trek toward the peak of your personal Glucotopia. Your journey, your pace.

Listening to your body is a crucial aspect of this journey. Your body communicates with you constantly, providing subtle clues about what it needs and how it's responding to your lifestyle changes. Pay attention to these signals. How do you feel after eating certain foods? Do you feel energized or sluggish after your morning workout? Are you waking up refreshed or tired? These valuable insights can guide your decisions and help you tailor the HAPPINESS principles to suit your unique needs and lifestyle.

Remember to celebrate your victories, big and small, along the way. Every time you choose a salad over a burger, meditate for five minutes, or get an extra hour of sleep, you're making progress. Celebrate these moments. These milestones, no matter how small they might seem, are stepping stones toward your bigger goals. They're proof of your commitment to your health and happiness.

Setbacks are not roadblocks on this journey; they're opportunities for learning and growth. Did you skip your workout or indulge in a high-sugar treat? Instead of being hard on yourself, use these instances to understand what led to them. Were you stressed? Did you not get enough sleep? Understanding these triggers can help you better manage such situations in the future.

Remember, you are not alone in this journey. Reach out to your loved ones, your health-care providers, or the communities around you for support and guidance. Sharing your journey can provide motivation, fresh perspectives, and much-needed support.

As we venture toward the culmination of this comprehensive guide, it's time to gaze into the future and to envision your Glucotopia—your idyllic state of health, happiness, and fulfillment. Everyone's Glucotopia will look different, shaped by their unique aspirations, circumstances, and visions of well-being.

Your Glucotopia could be a place where you're free of the physical and emotional burdens of diabetes, where you have the energy to pursue your passions, where you find joy in nourishing your body with wholesome food, or where peace and contentment are your constant companions. No matter what your Glucotopia looks like, it is a testament to your potential and the fulfilling life that lies ahead.

Setting realistic and achievable goals is the first step toward your Glucotopia. Break down your overarching objective into smaller, manageable targets. For instance, if your goal is to lose weight, start with a small target, perhaps losing 5 pounds in the next two months. If you wish to control your blood sugar levels, aim to reduce your HbA1c by 0.5% in the next six months. By setting attainable goals, you set yourself up for success, and each achievement fuels your motivation to reach the next milestone.

Remember, the journey to Glucotopia is not a sprint, but a marathon. It requires patience, persistence, and resilience. Embrace the process and give yourself grace and time to adapt to new habits. Lasting change does not happen overnight, but with consistent effort, you'll gradually start noticing the positive transformations in your health and well-being.

While it's important to strive for progress, it's equally important to acknowledge and accept that there will be ups and downs on this journey. There will be days when you feel motivated and empowered, and there will be days when things don't go as planned. And that's okay. Each day is a new opportunity to align yourself with your vision of Glucotopia.

As we turn the page to a new chapter in your health journey, remember that this journey is a testament to your strength, your courage, and your commitment to your health and happiness. You've embarked on a path that requires effort and dedication, but the destination—your Glucotopia—is well worth it.

As you continue on this journey, keep your eyes on the horizon, your Glucotopia gleaming in the distance. Step by step, with the

HAPPINESS formula as your guiding star, you're inching closer to a healthier, happier you.

As we reach the end of this enlightening journey, I want to acknowledge your commitment, curiosity, and courage. You have taken the first step toward a healthier, happier you. You have embraced the principles of the HAPPINESS formula and are ready to incorporate them into your daily life. Remember, this is not the end, but rather the beginning of a lifelong journey toward your very own Glucotopia.

The principles of the HAPPINESS formula are not merely guidelines; they represent a philosophy of living, a commitment to your health, happiness, and overall well-being. As you close this book, remember that the true power of this formula lies in its application. Embrace it as a part of your daily life and let it guide you toward your ideal state of health and happiness.

As you continue your journey, remember to celebrate each step you take, no matter how small. Be patient with yourself, trust in the process, and never lose sight of your goals. Remember, it's not about perfection, but about making consistent progress toward better health and happiness.

And so, I leave you with a promise of health, happiness, and a life transformed. May the principles of the HAPPINESS formula illuminate your path, and may you find joy in every step of your journey.

Thank you for joining me on this transformative journey through Glucotopia. Here's to your health, your happiness, and your incredible journey ahead. Your adventure is just beginning, and I am excited to see where it will take you.

Remember, you are not alone in this journey. We are a community bound by our shared commitment to health and happiness. And together, we will transform our lives, one day at a time, one step at a time, guided by the beacon of the HAPPINESS formula.

Until we meet again, stay strong, stay motivated, and above all, stay happy!

Here's to your journey,

Tabish Gill

References

Albosta, M., & Bakke, J. (2021). Intermittent fasting: is there a role in the treatment of diabetes? A review of the literature and guide for primary care physicians. *Clinical Diabetes & Endocrinology, 7*(1):3. https://www.ncbi.nlm.nih.gov/pmc/articles/PMC7856758/

American Diabetes Association. (n.d.). *Weekly exercise targets.* https://diabetes.org/healthy-living/fitness/weekly-exercise-targets

Anderson, R. C., Cookson, A. L., McNabb, W. C., Park, Z., McCann, M. J., Kelly, W. J., & Roy, N. C. (2010). *Lactobacillus plantarum MB452* enhances the function of the intestinal barrier by increasing the expression levels of genes involved in tight junction formation. *BMC Microbiology, 10*, 316. https://bmcmicrobiol.biomedcentral.com/articles/10.1186/1471-2180-10-316

Arnason, T. G., Bowen, M. W., & Mansell, K.D. (2017). Effects of intermittent fasting on health markers in those with type 2 diabetes: A pilot study. *World Journal of Diabetes, 8*(4):154-164. https://www.ncbi.nlm.nih.gov/pmc/articles/PMC5394735/

Bazzano, L. A., Li, T. Y., Joshipura, K. J., & Hu, F. B. (2008). Intake of fruit, vegetables, and fruit juices and risk of diabetes in women. *Diabetes Care, 31*(7), 1311–1317.

Bischoff, S. C., Barbara, G., Buurman, W., Ockhuizen, T., Schulzke, J.-D., Serino, M., Tilg, H., Watson, A., & Wells, J. M. (2014). Intestinal permeability – a new target for disease prevention and therapy. *BMC Gastroenterology, 14*, 189.

Black, D. S., & Slavich, G. (2016). Mindfulness meditation and the immune system: a systematic review of randomized controlled trials. *Annals of the New York Academy of Sciences, 1373*(1).

Blough, B., Moreland, A., & Mora, A., Jr. (2015). Metformin-induced lactic acidosis with emphasis on the anion gap. *Baylor University Medical Centre Proceedings, 28*(1), 31–33.

Camps, G., Mars, M., de Graaf, C., & Smeets, P. A. (2016). Empty calories and phantom fullness: a randomized trial studying the relative effects of energy density and viscosity on gastric emptying determined by MRI and satiety. *American Journal of Clinical Nutrition, 104*(1), 73–80.

Center for Drug Evaluation and Research. (2022, August 9). *FDA works to avoid shortage of sitagliptin following detection of nitrosamine impurity.* U.S. Food and Drug Administration. https://www.fda.gov/drugs/drug-safety-and-availability/fda-works-avoid-shortage-sitagliptin-following-detection-nitrosamine-impurity

Centers for Disease Control and Prevention. (2023, May 15). *Heart disease facts.* https://www.cdc.gov/heartdisease/facts.htm

Chevinsky, J. D., Wadden, T. A., & Chao, A. M. (2020). Binge eating disorder in patients with type 2 diabetes: Diagnostic and management challenges. *Diabetes, Metabolic Syndrome and Obesity, 13*, 1117–1131.

Chowdhury, R., Warnakula, S., Kunutsor, S., Crowe, F., Ward, H. A., Johnson, L., & Di Angelantonio, E. (2014). Association of dietary, circulating, and supplement fatty acids with coronary risk: a systematic review and meta-analysis. *Annals of Internal Medicine, 160*(6), 398–406.

Church, T. S., Blair, S. N., & Cocreham, S. (2010). Effects of Aerobic and resistance training on hemoglobin A1c Levels in patients with type 2 diabetes: A randomized controlled trial. *JAMA, 304*(20):2253–2262.

Colberg, S. R., Sigal, R. J., Yardley, J. E., Riddell, M. C., Dunstan, D. W., Dempsey, P. C., Horton, E. S., Castorino, K., & Tate, D. F. (2016). physical activity/exercise and diabetes: A position statement of the American Diabetes Association. *Diabetes Care, 39*(11), 2065–2079.

Cordain, L., Toohey, L., Smith, M. J., & Hickey, M. S. (2000). Modulation of immune function by dietary lectins in rheumatoid arthritis. *British Journal of Nutrition, 83*(3), 207–217.

Cummings, J. H., & Engineer, A. (2021). Denis Burkitt and the origins of the dietary fibre hypothesis. *Nutrition Research Reviews, 34*(1), 1–15.

Daley, C. A., Abbott, A., Doyle, P. S, Nader, G. A., Larson, S. (2010). A review of fatty acid profiles and antioxidant content in grass-fed and grain-fed beef. *Nutrition Journal, 9*, 10.

de Punder, K., & Pruimboon, L. (2013). The dietary intake of wheat and other cereal grains and their role in inflammation. *Nutrients, 5*(3), 771–787.

Diamanti-Kandarakis, E., & Dunaif, A. (2012). Insulin resistance and the polycystic ovary syndrome revisited: An update on mechanisms and implications. *Endocrine Reviews, 33*(6), 981–1030.

Duffey, K. J., & Popkin, B. M. (2011). Energy density, portion size, and eating occasions: contributions to increased energy intake in the United States, 1977–2006. *PLOS Medicine.*

Fasano, A. (2012). Leaky gut and autoimmune diseases. *Clinical Reviews in Allergy & Immunology, 42*(1), 71–78.

Fazzino, T. L., Rohde, K., & Sullivan, D. K. (2019), Hyper-palatable foods: Development of a quantitative definition and application to the US Food System Database. *Obesity, 27*, 1761–1768.

Fernan, C., Schult, J. P., & Niederdeppe, J. (2018). Health halo effects from product titles and nutrient content claims in the context of "protein" bars. *Health Communication, 33*(12), 1425–1433.

Francois, M. E., Baldi, J. C., Manning, P. J., Lucas, S. J. E., Hawley, J. A., Williams, M. J. A., & Cotter, J. D. (2014). 'Exercise snacks' before meals: A novel strategy to improve glycaemic control in individuals with insulin resistance. *Diabetologia,57*, 1437–1445.

Freed, D. L. (1991). Do dietary lectins cause disease? *BMJ, 318*(7190), 1023–1024.

Fung, J. (2016). *The obesity code: Unlocking the secrets of weight loss*. Greystone Books.

Gong, T., Wang, X., Yang, Y., Yan, Y., Yu, C., Zhou, R., & Jiang, W. (2017). Plant lectins activate the NLRP3 inflammasome to promote inflammatory disorders. *Journal of Immunology, 198*(5), 2082–2092.

Gundry, S. R. (2017). *The plant paradox: The hidden dangers in "healthy" foods that cause disease and weight gain*. Harper Wave.

Hajar, R. (2017). Risk factors for coronary artery disease: Historical perspectives. *Heart Views, 18*(3), 109–114.

Harvard T. H. Chan School of Public Health. (n.d.). *Lectins*. htt ps://www.hsph.harvard.edu/nutritionsource/anti-nutrients/lectins/

Hogan, S. (2017). Potential health hazards of eating red meat. *Journal of Internal Medicine, 281*(2), 106–122.

Hollander, D., Vadheim, C. M., Brettholz, E., Petersen, G. M., Delahunty, T., & Rotter, J. I. (1986). Increased intestinal permeability in patients with Crohn's disease and their relatives. *Annals of Internal Medicine, 105*(6), 883–885.

Hou, K., Wu, Z.-X., Chen, X.-Y., Wang, J.-Q., Zhang, D., Xiao, C., Zhu, D., Koya, J. B., Wei, L., Li, J., & Chen, Z.-S. (2022). Microbiota in health and diseases. *Signal Transduction and Targeted Therapy, 7*, 135.

Karsten, H., Patterson, P., Stout, R., & Crews, G. (2010). Vitamins A, E and fatty acid composition of the eggs of caged hens and pastured hens. *Renewable Agriculture and Food Systems*, 25(1), 45–54.

Kelley, D. E., He, J., Menshikova, E. V., & Ritov, V. B. (2002). Dysfunction of mitochondria in human skeletal muscle in type 2 diabetes. *Diabetes, 51*(10), 2944–50.

Kirwan, J. P., Sacks, J., & Nieuwoudt, S. (2017). The essential role of exercise in the management of type 2 diabetes. *Cleveland Clinic Journal of Medicine, 84*(7 Suppl. 1), S15–S21.

Krans, B. (2019, July 19). *Read the label: Your child's baby food may have too much sugar*. Healthline. https://www.healthline.com/health-news/how-you-can-tell-if -your-childs-baby-food-has-too-much-sugar

Lee, D., Albenberg, L., Compher, C., Baldassano, R., Piccoli, D .,Lewis, J. D., & Wu, G. D. (2015). Diet in the pathogenesis and treatment of inflammatory bowel diseases. *Gastroenterology, 148*(6), 1087–1106.

Lee, Y.M., Jacobs, D. R., Jr., & Lee, D. H. (2018). Persistent organic pollutants and type 2 diabetes: A critical review of review articles. *Frontiers in Endocrinology, 9*, 712.

Liener, I. E. (1994). Implications of antinutritional components in soybean foods. *Critical Reviews in Food Science and Nutrition, 34*(1), 31–67.

Lingappa N., & Mayrovitz, H. N. (2022). Role of sirtuins in diabetes and age-related processes. *Cureus, 14*(9), e28774.

Lovejoy, J. C. (2002). The influence of dietary fat on insulin resistance. *Current Diabetes Reports*, *2*, 435–440.

Malik, V. S., & Hu, F. B. (2015). Fructose and cardiometabolic health: What the evidence from sugar-sweetened beverages tells us. *Journal of the American College of Cardiology, 66*(14), 1615–1624.

McCarthy, M. I., & Zeggini, E. (2009). Genome-wide association studies in type 2 diabetes. *Current Diabetes Reports*, *9*(2), 164–171.

Medicines and Healthcare products Regulatory Agency. (2022, June 20). *Metformin and reduced vitamin B12 levels: New advice for monitoring patients at risk*. https://www.gov.uk/drug-safety-update/metformin-and-reduced-vitamin-b12-levels-new-advice-for-monitoring-patients-at-risk

Meng, Y., Li, S., Khan, J., Dai, Z., Li, C., Hu, X., Shen, Q., & Xue, Y. (2021). Sugar- and artificially sweetened beverages consumption linked to type 2 diabetes, cardiovascular diseases, and all-cause mortality: A systematic review and dose-response meta-analysis of prospective cohort studies. *Nutrients*, 13(8), 2636.

Mkumbuzi, L., Mfengu, M. M. O. , Engwa, G. A., & Sewani-Rusike, C. R. (2020). Insulin resistance is associated with gut permeability without the direct influence of obesity in young adults. *Diabetes, Metabolic Syndrome and Obesity*, *13*, 2997–3008.

Mohammed, S. (2021, August 31). *The '10-3-2-1-0 formula' can help you sleep better and wake up in the morning feeling refreshed, and it's dead simple.* Glamour. https://www.glamourmagazine.co.uk/article/10-3-2-1-0-sleep-formula

Moss, M. (2014). *Salt, sugar, fat: How the food giants hooked us*. WH Allen.

Ortolan, S., Neunhaeuserer, D., Quinto, G., Barra, B., Centanini, A., Battista, F., Vecchiato, M., De Marchi, V., Celidoni, M., Rebba, V., & Ermolao, A. (2022). Potential cost savings for the healthcare system by physical activity in different chronic diseases: A pilot study in the Veneto region of Italy. *International Journal of Environmental Research and Public Health, 19*(12), 7375.

Rolls, B. J., Morris, E. L., & Roe, L.S. (2002). Portion size of food affects energy intake in normal-weight and overweight men and women. *American Journal of Clinical Nutrition*, *76*(6), 120–13.

Savage, D. B., Petersen, K. F., & Shulman, G. I. Mechanisms of insulin resistance in humans and possible links with inflammation. *Hypertension*, *45*(5), 828–33.

Selhub, E. M., Logan, A. C., & Bested, A. C. (2014). Fermented foods, microbiota, and mental health: ancient practice meets nutritional psychiatry. *Journal of Physiological Anthropology*, *33*(1), 2.

Seven Countries Study. (2020, February 11). https://www.sevenc ountriesstudy.com/

Sharon, N. (2007). Lectins: carbohydrate-specific reagents and biological recognition molecules. *Journal of Biological Chemistry*, *282*(5), 2753–2764.

Siri-Tarino, P. W., Sun, Q., Hu, F. B., & Krauss, R. M. (2010). Meta-analysis of prospective cohort studies evaluating the association of saturated fat with cardiovascular disease. *The American Journal of Clinical Nutrition*, *91*(3), 535–546.

Takiishi, T., Fenero, C. I. M., & Câmera, N. O. S. (2017). Intestinal barrier and gut microbiota: Shaping our immune responses throughout life. *Tissue Barriers*, *5*(4): e1373208.

van der Velde, J. H. P. M., Boone, S. C., Winters-van Eekelen, E., Hesselink, M. K. C., Schrauwen-Hinderling, V. B., Schrauwen, P., Lamb, H. J., Rosendaal, F. R., & de Mutsert, R. (2023). Timing of physical activity in relation to liver fat content and insulin resistance. *Diabetologia*, *66*, 461–471.

Vasconcelos, I. M., & Oliveira, J. T. (2004). Antinutritional properties of plant lectins. *Toxicon*, *44*(4), 385–403.

Vidali, S., Aminzadeh, S., Lambert, B., Rutherford, T., Sperl, W., Kofler, B., & Feichtinger, R. G. (2015). Mitochondria: The ketogenic diet—A metabolism-based therapy, *The International Journal of Biochemistry & Cell Biology*, *63*, 55–59.

Vojdani, A., & Tarash, I. (2013). Cross-reaction between gliadin and different food and tissue antigens. *Food and Nutrition Sciences*, *4*(1), 20–32.

World Health Organization. (2015, March 4). *WHO calls on countries to reduce sugars intake among adults and children*. https://www.who.int/news/item/04-03-2015-who-calls-on-c ountries-to-reduce-sugars-intake-among-adults-and-children

World Health Organization. (2020, March 4). *Obesity and its roots*. https://www.who.int/news-room/events/detail/2020/03/04/default-calendar/world-obesity-day

Yao, S., Zhao, Z., Wang, W., & Liu, X. (2021). *Bifidobacterium longum*: Protection against inflammatory bowel disease. *Journal of Immunology Research*, *2021*: 8030297.

Young, L. R, & Nestle, M. (2002). The contribution of expanding portion sizes to the us obesity epidemic. *American Journal of Public Health*, *92*(2), 246–249.

Zhang, K., Bai, P., & Deng, Z. (2021). Dose-Dependent Effect of Intake of Fermented Dairy Foods on the Risk of Diabetes: Results From a Meta-analysis. *Canadian Journal of Diabetes*, 46(3). https://www.canadianjournalofdiabetes.com/article/S1499-2671(21)00247-1/fulltext

Zheng, Y., Zhang, Z., Tang, P., Wu, Y., Zhang, A., Li, D., Wang, C.-Z., Wan, J.-Y., Yao, H., & Yuan, C.-S. (2023). Probiotics Fortify Intestinal Barrier Function: A Systematic Review and Meta-Analysis of Randomized Trials. *Journal Name*, *Volume Number*, *Page Range*. https://www.frontiersin.org/articles/10.3389/fimmu.2023.1143548/full

www.ingramcontent.com/pod-product-compliance
Lightning Source LLC
Chambersburg PA
CBHW031539260326
41914CB00002B/197